ECGs for the
Emergency Physician 2

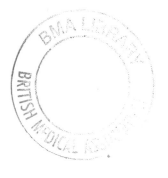
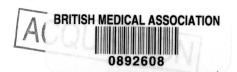

ECGs for the Emergency Physician 2

Amal Mattu

Director, Emergency Medicine Residency Program, Associate Professor, Department of Emergency Medicine, University of Maryland School of Medicine, Baltimore, Maryland, USA

William Brady

Professor and Vice Chair, Department of Emergency Medicine, and Professor, Department of Internal Medicine, University of Virginia School of Medicine, Charlottesville, Virginia, USA

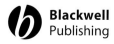
Blackwell
Publishing

© 2008 Amal Mattu & William Brady
Published by Blackwell Publishing
BMJ Books is an imprint of the BMJ Publishing Group Limited, used under licence
Blackwell Publishing, Inc., 350 Main Street, Malden, Massachusetts 02148-5020, USA
Blackwell Publishing Ltd, 9600 Garsington Road, Oxford OX4 2DQ, UK
Blackwell Publishing Asia Pty Ltd, 550 Swanston Street, Carlton, Victoria 3053, Australia

The right of the Author to be identified as the Author of this Work has been asserted in accordance
with the Copyright, Designs and Patents Act 1988.

First published 2008
1   2008

Library of Congress Cataloging-in-Publication Data
Mattu, Amal.
    ECGs for the emergency physician 2 / Amal Mattu, William Brady.
        p. ; cm.
    "BMJ Books."
    Includes index.
    ISBN 978-1-4051-5701-8 (pbk. : alk. paper)   1. Electrocardiography.   2. Emergency physicians.
I. Brady, William, 1960-   II. Title.
    [DNLM: 1. Electrocardiography—methods.   2. Emergency Medical Services.   3. Heart Diseases—diagnosis.
WG 140 M444e 2007]
    RC683.5.E5M344 2007
    616.1′207547—dc22   2007025971

A catalogue record for this title is available from the British Library

Set in 9/13 pt Frutiger by Graphicraft Limited, Hong Kong
Printed and bound in Singapore by C.O.S. Printers Pte Ltd

Commissioning Editor: Mary Banks
Development Editor: Lauren Brindley
Production Controller: Rachel Edwards

For further information on Blackwell Publishing, visit our website:
http://www.blackwellpublishing.com

The publisher's policy is to use permanent paper from mills that operate a sustainable forestry policy, and which has
been manufactured from pulp processed using acid-free and elementary chlorine-free practices. Furthermore, the publisher
ensures that the text paper and cover board used have met acceptable environmental accreditation standards.

Contents

Foreword vii

Preface ix

Dedications xi

Part 1   Focus on dysrhythmias

Case histories 3

ECG interpretations and comments 17

Part 2   12-Lead ECGs (intermediate level)

Case histories 29

ECG interpretations and comments 78

Part 3   12-Lead ECGs (advanced level)

Case histories 119

ECG interpretations and comments 164

Appendix A: Differential diagnoses 203

Appendix B: Commonly used abbreviations 205

Index 207

Foreword

Do you remember that patient you sent home? It is said that nothing good ever follows that question. One of the most dreaded scenarios is the case where an ECG was misinterpreted, or where the diagnosis, now evident on the ECG, was missed, and the patient was inadvertently (and inappropriately), sent home. How has the ECG become so important to the practice of medicine in the emergency department?

An electrocardiogram (ECG or EKG, abbreviated from the German Elektrokardiogramm) is a graphic produced by an electrocardiograph, which records the electrical activity of the heart over time. In 1902, Willem Einthoven, working in Leiden, The Netherlands, used a galvanometer to record the electrical activity of the heart over time.[1] Einthoven assigned the letters P, Q, R, S and T to the various deflections, and described the electrocardiographic findings for a number of disease states. In 1924, he was awarded the Nobel Prize in Medicine for his discovery.[2]

The ECG has become a fundamental adjunct to the physical exam, owing to its utility in the diagnosis of cardiac arrhythmias, acute myocardial infarction (MI), electrolyte imbalances such as hyperkalemia and hypokalemia, conduction abnormalities, ischemic heart disease and select non-cardiac diseases such as pulmonary embolism, hyperthyroidism and hypothermia.[3–5] While not considered a modern discovery, understanding of the clinical correlation of the ECG to a variety of disease states is undergoing continuous refinement. The ECG has become so familiar to the general population and is a prominent icon for the technology of medicine having been incorporated into the logos of many medical organizations.

Every medical student has personal reflections on how interpretation of the ECG was first learned. ECG and rhythm interpretation is one of the fundamental skills that are learned during clinical clerkships in medical school. For emergency physicians, ECGs are interpreted countless times per day, with these interpretations forming the basis for life saving decision-making. In emergency medicine, the ECG is emblematic of the potential for missed diagnosis, if, for example, the ECG is misinterpreted or simply not done.

ECGs have become such an essential part of emergency medicine that they are often performed before the patient can be fully evaluated by the physician. Further, the ECG is often performed even before the patient is transported to the hospital. With the emphasis of reduced time to reperfusion for patients with ST elevation MI, or STEMI, delays in ECG acquisition can have disastrous consequences; conversely, the early use of the ECG in the prehospital setting can markedly reduce the time to hospital-based reperfusion in STEMI.[6]

The authors, Drs. Mattu and Brady, are widely known for their work in the science and clinical application of ECGs in the emergency setting. Given the realities of the practice of emergency medicine, the authors of *ECGs for the Emergency Physician*, Volume 2, have chosen to recreate the clinical setting by presenting the tracing with the brief clinical history. The reader is asked to interpret the tracing in the first half of each section, and answers are given in the second half of the section, for readers to check accuracy and thoroughness. The tracings in this text thus become the essential teaching file for clinicians to use in acquiring the in-depth understanding needed by emergency physicians. This book contains a vast array of ECG tracings that duplicates the experience of clinical work by demonstrating the commonly encountered ECG abnormalities. Whether this text is used as a reference or a challenging exercise, the reader will be exposed to 200 classic ECGs with extensive descriptions of the salient clinical points associated with each. Much as the ECG interpretation is an essential skill in emergency medicine, this text is essential reading for the emergency physician.

Robert E. O'Connor, MD, MPH
Professor and Chair
Department of Emergency Medicine
University of Virginia Health System
Charlottesville, Virginia

References

1. Einthoven W. Un nouveau galvanometre. *Arch Neerl Sc Ex Nat* 1901;**6**:625.
2. Cooper JK. Electrocardiography 100 years ago. Origins, pioneers, and contributors. *New Engl J Med* 1986;**315**(7):461–4.
3. Braunwald E. (Ed) *Heart Disease: A Textbook of Cardiovascular Medicine*, 5th edn. Philadelphia: W.B. Saunders Co., 1997.
4. 2005 American Heart Association Guidelines for Cardiopulmonary Resuscitation and Emergency Cardiovascular Care—Part 8: Stabilization of the Patient With Acute Coronary Syndromes. *Circulation* 2005;**112**: IV-89– IV-110.
5. Van Mieghem C, Sabbe M, Knockaert D. The clinical value of the ECG in noncardiac conditions. *Chest* 2004;**125**(4):1561–76.
6. Henry TD, Sharkey SW, Burke MN, Chavez IJ, Graham KJ, Henry CR, Lips DL, Madison JD, Menssen KM, Mooney MR, Newell MC, Pedersen WR, Poulose AK, Traverse JH, Unger BT, Wang YL, Larson DM. A regional system to provide timely access to percutaneous coronary intervention for ST-elevation myocardial infarction. *Circulation* 2007;**116**(7):721–8.

Preface

The adult male with chest pain and diaphoresis... ...*ultimately diagnosed with STEMI*. The fussy infant with a very rapid pulse... ...*found to have Wolff-Parkinson-White syndrome-related PSVT*. The young adult female with altered mental status and a wide QRS complex... ...*demonstrating significant cardiovascular end-organ toxicity due to tricyclic antidepressant poisoning*. The elderly female "found down," pulseless and apneic... ...*presenting with a bradycardic PEA cardiac arrest rhythm*. The hypothermic patient with bradycardia... ...*as well as significant J waves*.

These clinical scenarios are quite familiar to the practicing emergency physician. In each presentation, the electrocardiogram (ECG) is a primary diagnostic tool used by the emergency physician in the early evaluation of these very ill patients. A significant number of the millions of patients cared for each year in emergency departments present with cardiovascular syndromes and/or issues related to the cardiovascular system. The widely recognized benefits of early diagnosis and rapid treatment of cardiovascular emergencies have only emphasized the importance of emergency physician competency in electrocardiographic interpretation. The emergency physician, frequently the first – if not the only – physician to evaluate such patients, is charged with the responsibility of rapid, accurate diagnosis followed by appropriate therapy delivered expeditiously. Emergency physicians are immediately available at all times of the day and night to care for patients with time-sensitive cardiovascular emergencies. This evaluation frequently involves the performance of and interpretation of the ECG. These interpretations often occur without the benefit of past knowledge of the patient, without the results of exhaustive prior evaluations, and without prior electrocardiograms for comparison – and usually in the midst of a busy, or even chaotic, emergency department environment.

Further emphasizing the importance of electrocardiography is the fact that it remains one of the most cost-effective and useful tests in medicine. It is inexpensive, rapid, and reliable. It can be performed at the bedside in the sickest of patients – by anyone with minimal training – often providing information that will make the difference between life and death. The knowledge to master this electrocardiography interpretation doesn't require any special type of residency or fellowship training, and it doesn't require thousands of dollars to be paid for travel and tuition at continuing medical education courses. *It can be learned from books.*

This text, *ECGs for the Emergency Physician 2*, continues with the case-based instruction and electrocardiographic experience that was so well-received in *ECGs for the Emergency Physician 1*. Like Volume 1, this Volume contains two hundred ECGs accompanied by brief, focused case histories. However, in response to the enthusiastic feedback from Volume 1, we have further increased the overall level of difficulty of the ECGs but without relying on esoterica – all cases are real emergency department presentations, the type that emergency physicians must always be ready to face. We've also added greater emphasis on dysrhythmias, including an initial section purely focused on dysrhythmia interpretation primarily from rhythms strips. Readers of Volume 1 enjoyed the pearls, pitfalls, and patient outcomes so we've added more. Readers expressed appreciation for the repetition of key points in the Commentary sections which helped emphasize important points, so we've maintained this. Readers also gave positive feedback regarding the use of illustrations in the Commentary section, so we've increased the use of explanatory illustrations as well. As with Volume 1, we continue to focus on teaching the intermediate and advanced-level practitioner, and thus there is no "basic" section or "introduction to ECG interpretation." Those readers that are new to the art of ECG interpretation are referred to the multitude of ECG books on the market that focus on beginners' skills.

Lastly, we'd like to emphasize that Volume 2 was not written as a *replacement* to, or alternative, to Volume 1 but rather as an *extension* of Volume 1. We strongly believe that although these two texts may be used individually, when used in combination they represent one of the most comprehensive and educational ECG collections ever assembled for emergency physicians and other acute health care providers. Our sincerest hope is that these books will help emergency physicians around the world to continue to save lives every day.

Amal Mattu and William Brady

Dedications

For my father, William J Brady, Sr, a good man.

William Brady

I would like to thank my wife, Sejal, for her constant support and patience; to my children Nikhil, Eleena, and Kamran for helping me keep balance in my life; to the faculty and residents of the University of Maryland Emergency Medicine Residency Program for their inspiration and for their ECG contributions; to Lauren Brindley and BMJ Books/Blackwell Publishing for supporting our work; to Dr. Bill Brady for his friendship, mentorship, and for being a true academic role model; and to emergency physicians around the world – your dedication to patient care and commitment to education are a constant source of inspiration and reminder of why I am so proud to be a member of this profession.

Amal Mattu

Part 1
Focus on dysrhythmias

Case histories

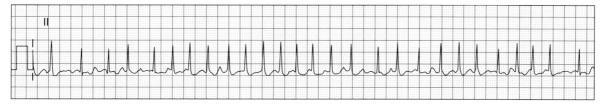

1. 63 year old woman with palpitations, weakness, and dyspnea

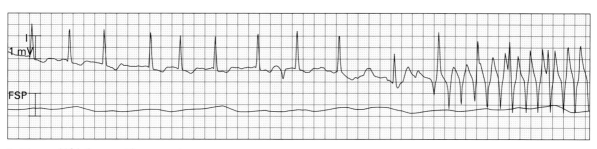

2. 71 year old febrile man with pneumonia

a)

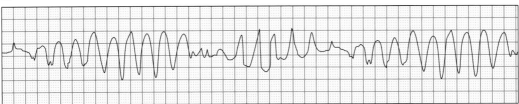

b)

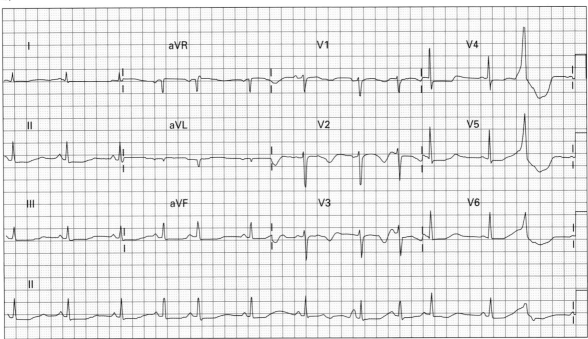

3. 54 year old dehydrated woman with gastroenteritis and recurrent syncope, a) during an episode of "syncope", b) after spontaneous conversion

a)

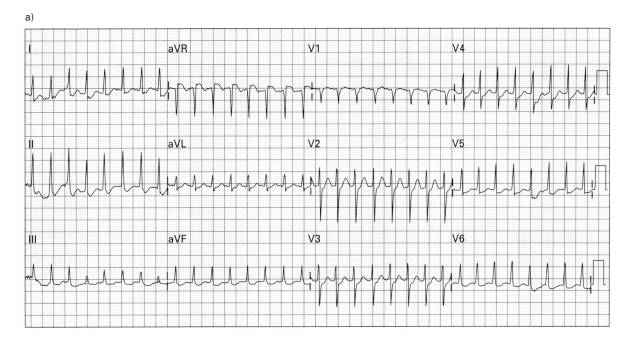

b)

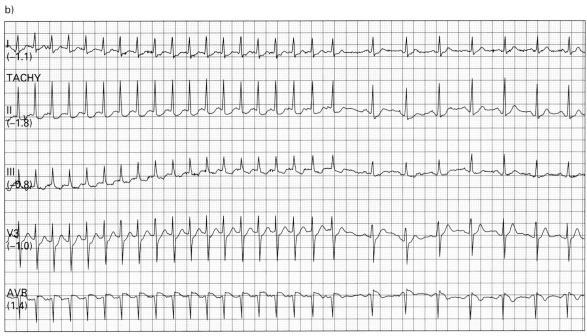

4. a) 18 year old woman with palpitations, dizziness, and hypotension, b) during treatment

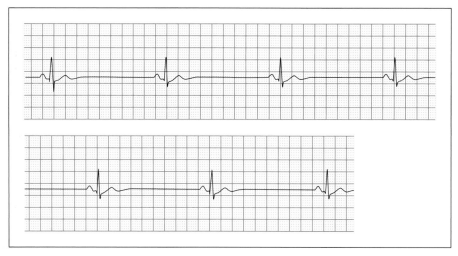

5. 68 year old man with hypertension, managed with three medications, presenting with profound weakness

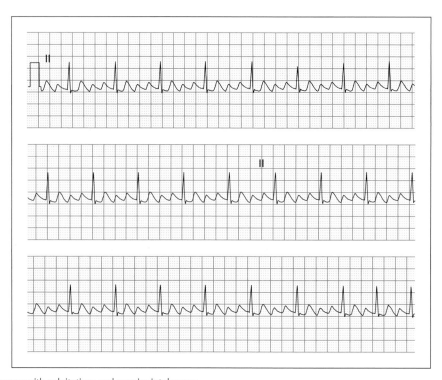

6. 57 year old woman with palpitations and exercise intolerance

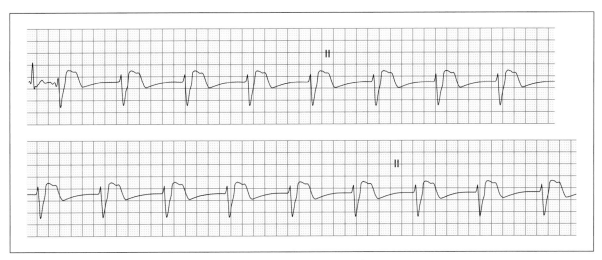

7. 42 year old man 30 minutes after receiving fibrinolytics for an acute myocardial infarction

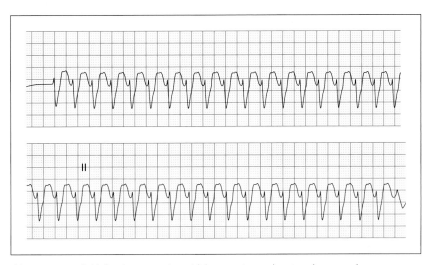

8. 53 year old man with past myocardial infarction presenting with hypotension and acute pulmonary edema

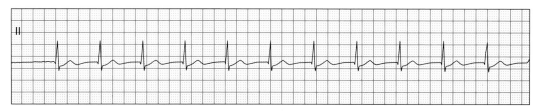

9. 79 year old woman with hypertension and chronic congestive heart failure complaining of weakness and dyspnea

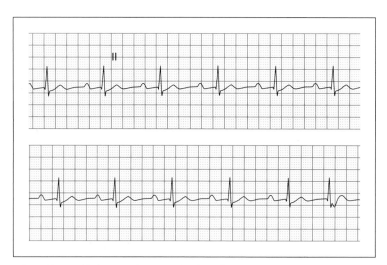

10. 29 year old man presenting with an ankle fracture; the patient is a long-distance runner

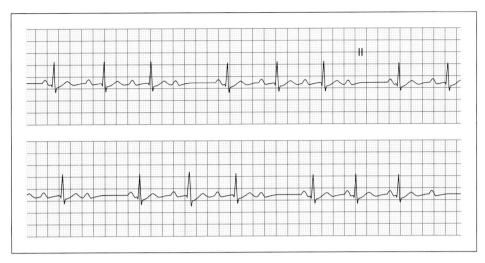

11. 71 year old woman with syncope

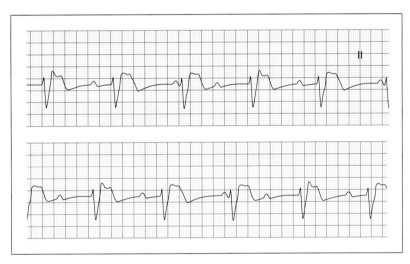

12. 79 year old man with progressive weakness

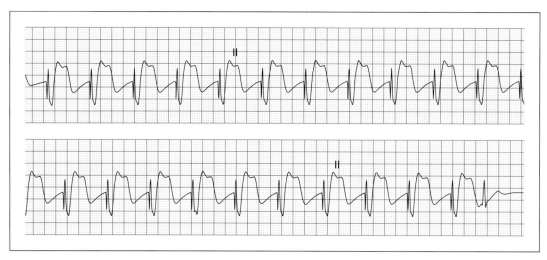

13. 59 year old woman being resuscitated during a cardiac arrest

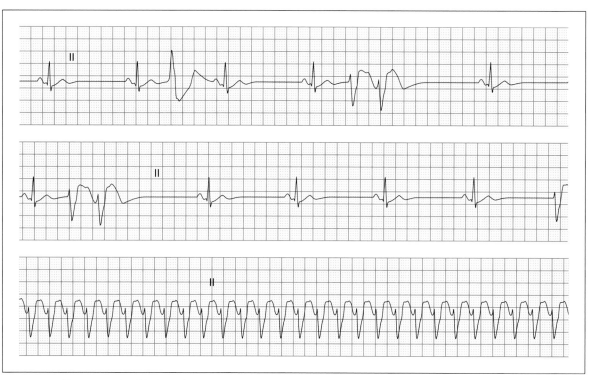

14. 68 year old woman with sudden loss of consciousness

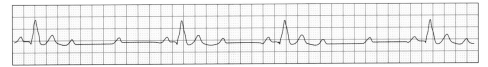

15. 66 year old man with a history of sick sinus syndrome and hypertension who notes extreme dizziness

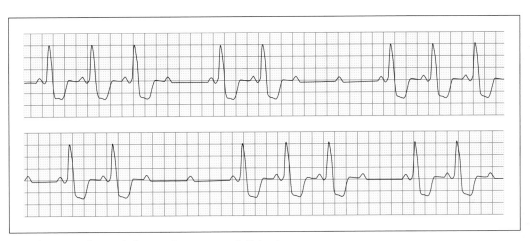

16. 56 year old woman with recently diagnosed acute myocardial infarction

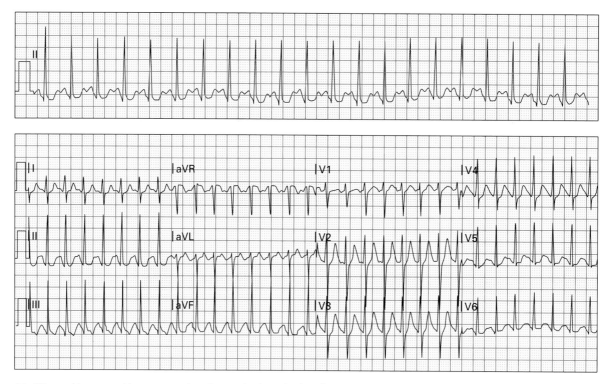

17. 26 year old woman with extreme anxiety after cocaine ingestion (nasal)

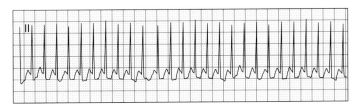

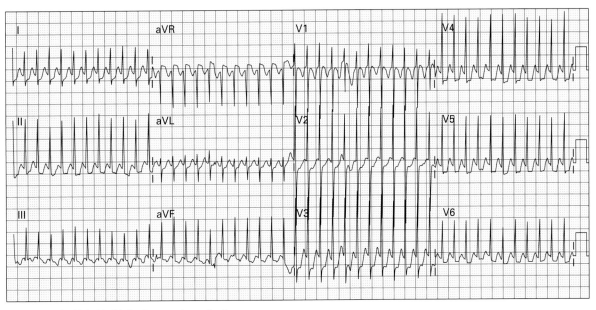

18. 18 month old child with fussiness and poor feeding

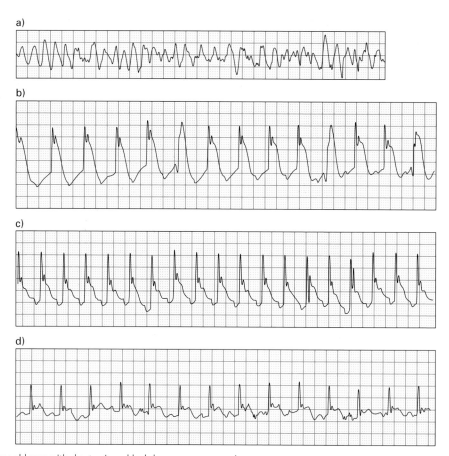

19. a)–d) 54 year old man with chest pain suddenly becomes unresponsive

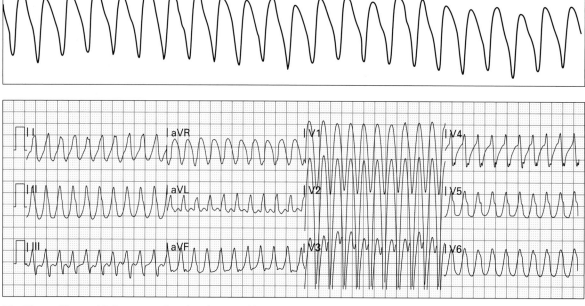

20. 60 year old man with dyspnea, profound weakness, and hypotension

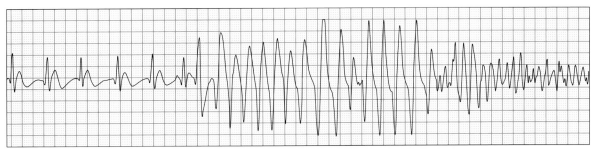

21. 65 year old woman with chest pain suspected of acute myocardial infarction and sudden loss of consciousness

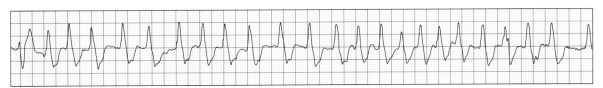

22. 67 year old woman with the sensation of a rapid heart beat

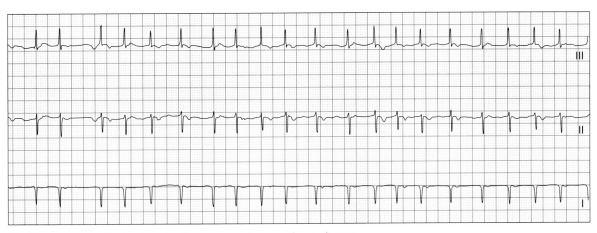

23. 65 year old man with chronic obstructive pulmonary disease and acute dyspnea

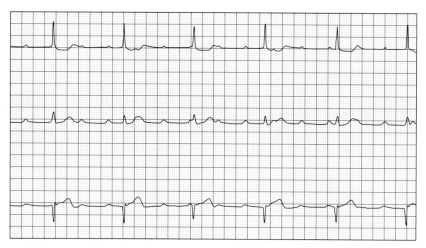

24. 75 year old woman with a decreased level of consciousness

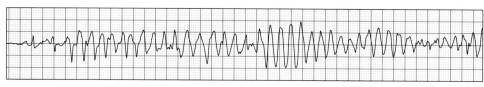

25. 16 year old boy presents after a syncopal episode, now with recurrent sudden loss of consciousness

ECG interpretations and comments

(Rates refer to ventricular rate unless otherwise indicated)

1. **Atrial fibrillation, ventricular rate 138.** The rhythm is a narrow QRS complex, irregularly irregular tachycardia. The differential diagnosis includes atrial fibrillation, atrial flutter with variable conduction, and multifocal atrial tachycardia (MAT). Given the absence of distinct P-waves or flutter waves, the diagnosis of atrial fibrillation is made.

2. **Atrial fibrillation, ventricular rate 96, artifact.** The rhythm is initially irregularly irregular without distinct atrial activity, consistent with atrial fibrillation. The rhythm terminates with an episode of markedly irregular and rapid QRS complexes with changing morphologies. Considerations with this type of rhythm should include atrial fibrillation with Wolff-Parkinson-White syndrome (WPW), torsades de pointes, or artifact. The presence of "sharp points" at *both* the apices and nadirs of the QRS complexes is more consistent with artifact. See figure below.

This figure corresponds to case #2. Atrial fibrillation with subsequent wide QRS complex tachycardia

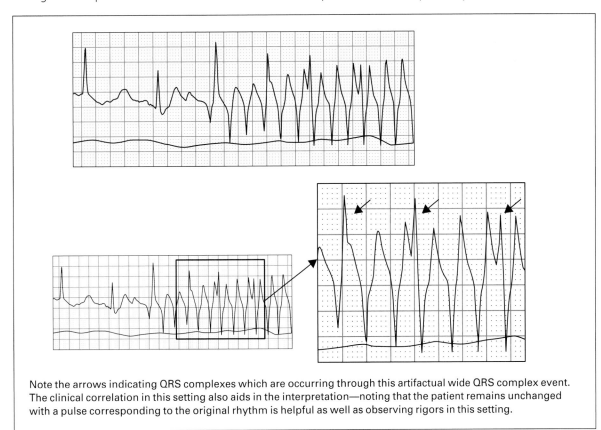

Note the arrows indicating QRS complexes which are occurring through this artifactual wide QRS complex event. The clinical correlation in this setting also aids in the interpretation—noting that the patient remains unchanged with a pulse corresponding to the original rhythm is helpful as well as observing rigors in this setting.

3. **a) Polymorphic ventricular tachycardia, suspected torsade de pointes, rate 220.** The rhythm is a wide QRS complex tachycardia with continuously varying QRS complex morphology, variation in the R-R intervals, and variation of the electrical axis consistent with polymorphic ventricular tachycardia. The QRS complexes appear to rotate around a fixed point, growing larger, then smaller, then larger, and so on. This pattern is suggestive of torsade de pointes. Torsade de pointes is a type of polymorphic ventricular tachycardia characterized by this unusual morphology. It is also defined when the baseline ECG demonstrates a prolonged QT-interval.

    b) Sinus rhythm (SR), rate 64, premature atrial contractions (PACs) and premature ventricular contractions (PVCs), anteroseptal ischemia, prolonged QT-interval. The major abnormality here is prolongation of the QT-interval. The normal QT-interval will vary based on rate, and so the Bazett formula is used to correct the QT-interval based on the rate: corrected QT (QTc) = QT/√(RR). RR represents the R-R interval. The QTc is considered prolonged when >450 msec in men and >460 msec in women and children. A prolonged QTc indicates that the patient is at risk for torsade de pointes. The major risk for this dysrhythmia appears to occur when the QTc is ≥500 msec.[1] In this case, there is marked prolongation (QT = 600 msec, QTc = 620 msec). The differential diagnosis of a prolonged QT-interval includes hypokalemia, hypomagnesemia, hypocalcemia, acute myocardial ischemia, elevated intracranial pressure, drugs with sodium channel blocking effects, hypothermia, and congenital prolonged QT syndrome. The QT-interval prolongation in this case (as well as the premature contractions) was caused by electrolyte abnormalities. T-wave inversions in leads V1–V3 suggest anteroseptal ischemia. See figure below.

This figure corresponds to case #3. Polymorphic ventricular tachycardia, torsade de pointes

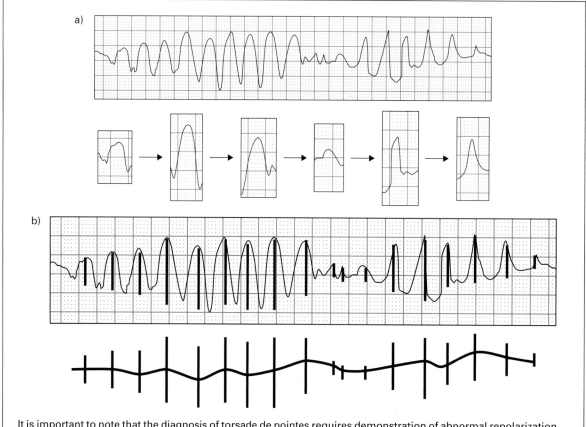

It is important to note that the diagnosis of torsade de pointes requires demonstration of abnormal repolarization on the ECG, namely prolongation of the QT-interval. a) Note the significant beat-to-beat variation in the QRS complex morphology. b) Note the significant beat-to-beat variation in the QRS complex amplitude.

4.   **a) Paroxysmal supraventricular tachycardia, rate 190.** The differential diagnosis of a regular, narrow QRS complex tachycardia includes sinus tachycardia (ST), paroxysmal supraventricular tachycardia (often simply referred to as supraventricular tachycardia, or SVT), and atrial flutter with 2:1 atrioventricular conduction. ST and atrial flutter are characterized by distinct atrial activity on the ECG. SVTs, on the other hand, often have absence of clear atrial activity or they may demonstrate retrograde P-waves (P-waves that occur just after the QRS complex, demonstrated in later cases). This ECG lacks obvious sinus P-waves or flutter waves, so the diagnosis of SVT is made. ST-segment depression is noted in the inferior and lateral leads, a common finding in cases of SVT and without clinical relevance as long as the ST-segment depression resolves after conversion to SR.
     b) Paroxysmal supraventricular tachycardia, rate 190, with conversion to sinus tachycardia, rate 105. This multi-lead rhythm strip was obtained during intravenous adenosine infusion. A brief pause is followed by a return to SR.

5.   **Sinus bradycardia (SB), rate 20.** A regular, narrow QRS complex bradycardia is present. A P-wave is associated with each QRS complex. The intrinsic rate of the sinus node is 60–100 beats/minute. When the sinus rate is <60 beats/minute, it is referred to as sinus bradycardia.

6.   **Atrial flutter with 4:1 atrioventricular (AV) conduction, rate 75.** A regular, narrow QRS complex rhythm is present. Regular atrial activity is noted at a rate of 300 beats/minute (every 4th complex is hidden within a QRS complex) and produces a "saw-tooth" pattern typical of flutter waves between the QRS complexes. The ventricular response rate is one-quarter the atrial rate, consistent with a 4:1 AV conduction ratio. See figure below.

This figure corresponds to case #6. Atrial flutter

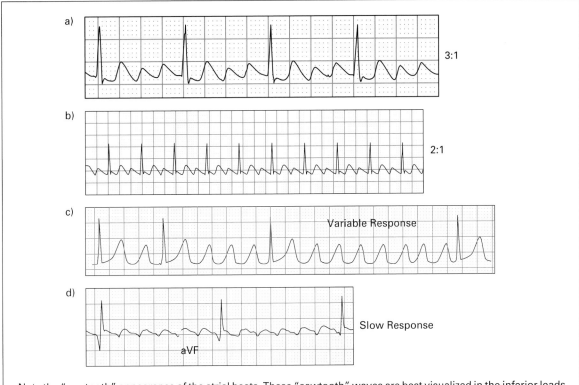

Note the "sawtooth" appearance of the atrial beats. These "sawtooth" waves are best visualized in the inferior leads (II, III, and aVF) and V1. The ventricular response ranges from slow to rapid with both regular and irregular response. The response is best expressed as a function of the number of P-waves relative to the QRS complex that ultimately results from a conducted impulse. a) 3:1 conduction. b) 2:1 conduction. Note that a ventricular rate of 150/minute should always prompt consideration of atrial flutter. c) Variable, or irregular, response. d) Slow response.

7. **Accelerated idioventricular rhythm, rate 55.** A regular, wide QRS complex rhythm is noted. No P-waves are present, ruling out an atrial origin for the beats. The likely rhythm, then, is ventricular. Because the normal ventricular escape rate is 20–40 beats/minute, this rhythm is termed an *accelerated* ventricular escape rhythm or accelerated idioventricular rhythm. This type of rhythm is commonly noted in patients with acute MI who spontaneously or therapeutically reperfuse. A junctional rhythm with aberrant ventricular conduction (e.g. bundle branch block) is also capable of producing a regular wide QRS complex rhythm at this rate and without P-waves; however, the QRS morphologies are not typical for the presence of either a left or right bundle branch block. A full 12-lead ECG would be helpful for clarification.

8. **Probable ventricular tachycardia (VT), rate 170.** The differential diagnosis of a regular, wide QRS complex tachydysrhythmia includes ST with aberrant conduction (e.g. bundle branch block), SVT or atrial flutter with aberrant ventricular conduction, and VT. Neither P-waves nor flutter waves are found, leaving SVT with aberrant ventricular conduction and VT as the two main diagnostic possibilities. Without any clinical information, it is estimated that >80% of the time these rhythms are confirmed as VT. Given the additional clinical information of the patient's-age, past MI, hypotension, and acute pulmonary edema, however, the certainty of VT is nearly 100%. See figure opposite.

9. **Accelerated AV junctional rhythm, rate 80.** The QRS complexes are narrow and there are no P-waves noted, ruling out a ventricular rhythm and atrial rhythm, respectively. Narrow QRS complex rhythms of this type are likely to originate in the AV node. Because the intrinsic pacing rate of the AV node is 40–60 beats/minute, the rhythm is termed an *accelerated* AV junctional rhythm.

10. **SR with first degree AV block, rate 60, premature junctional complex (PJC) with aberrant conduction.** The rhythm has narrow QRS complexes which, with exception of the last QRS complex, are all followed by P-waves. The PR-intervals are constant and prolonged (320 msec; normal = 120–200 msec), diagnostic of a first degree AV block. The last QRS complex is a PJC with slight aberrant conduction: it appears early in the cycle, it is not preceded by a P-wave, and it has a similar morphology to the earlier QRS complexes except for some slight aberrancy of the terminal portion of the S-wave.

11. **SR with second degree AV block type 1 (Wenckebach, Mobitz I), rate 60.** The P-waves are constant and are noted preceding each of the QRS complexes. However, some P-waves are non-conducted and instead followed by a pause. The PR-intervals demonstrate gradual elongation before each non-conducted P-wave. This pattern is typical of SR with second degree AV block type 1, also known as Wenckebach or Mobitz I AV conduction. See figure opposite.

12. **SR with AV dissociation and third degree AV block, accelerated idioventricular rhythm, rate 50.** A regular, wide QRS complex bradycardia is present. Regularly occurring P waves are also noted at a different rate than the QRS complexes, suggesting independent atrial and ventricular activity (AV dissociation). There is no evidence that any of the P-waves are being conducted to the ventricle (third degree AV block). QRS complexes are wide (>120 msec) and appear to be ventricular in origin. Because the rate of this ventricular escape rhythm, or "idioventricular rhythm," is faster than the intrinsic pacing rate of the ventricle (20–40 beats/minute), accelerated idioventricular rhythm is diagnosed. See figure on p. 22.

13. **100% ventricular paced rhythm, rate 70.** Narrow pacemaker stimuli ("spikes") appear just before each QRS complex. There is no evidence of independent atrial or ventricular activity. The QRS compexes are wide, typical of artificially paced rhythms. See figure on p. 22.

This figure corresponds to case #8

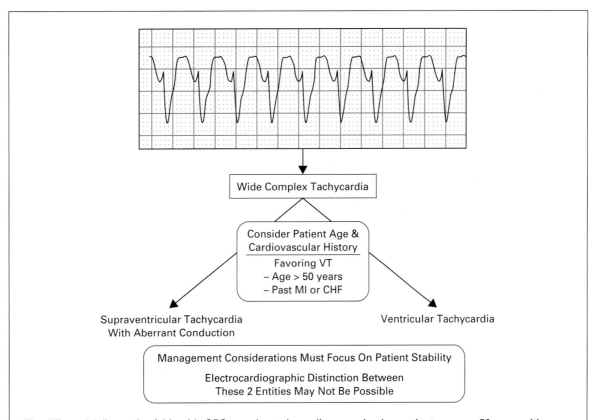

The differential diagnosis of this wide QRS complex tachycardia, occurring in a patient over age 50 years with a past history of MI, includes both supraventricular tachycardia (SVT) with aberrant conduction and ventricular tachycardia (VT). Clinical history, such as past MI and congestive heart failure, strongly suggest VT. Useful electrocardiographic findings suggestive of VT include AV dissociation, fusion and capture beats, and concordancy of the precordial QRS complexes. Nonetheless, the distinction of VT from SVT based on clinical and electrocardiographic criteria may not be possible. Management decisions should include clinical and ECG information yet must focus on stability. Markers of instability include hypotension or hypoperfusion, dyspnea due to pulmonary edema, chest pain due to coronary ischemia, and depressed mental status.

This figure corresponds to case #11. Second degree AV block type 1

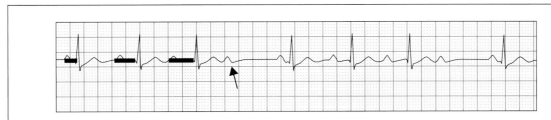

Observe the relationship between the P-wave and QRS complex, characterized by progressively longer PR interval with ultimate dropped beat as noted by the arrow (i.e., no QRS complex). The QRS complex is narrow. Group beating, or a clustering of QRS complexes, is seen as well.

This figure corresponds to case #12. Third degree, or complete, AV block

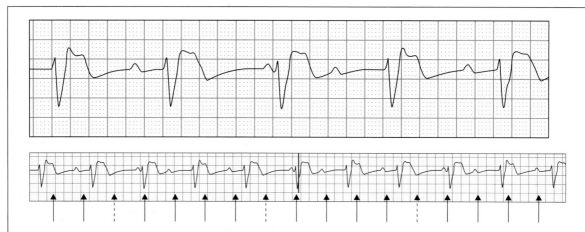

Note the occurrence of P-waves and QRS complexes which are independent of one another. The atrial rate, as signified by the P-waves (solid arrows), is more rapid than the ventricular rate (the QRS complexes). The P-waves are occurring at a rate of approximately 110/minute while the QRS complexes are at a rate of approximately 50/minute. Note that certain P-waves may be lost (dotted arrow), or obscured, by certain portions of the QRS complex. The QRS complex is usually widened in third degree heart block.

This figure corresponds to case #13. Electronic ventricular paced rhythm

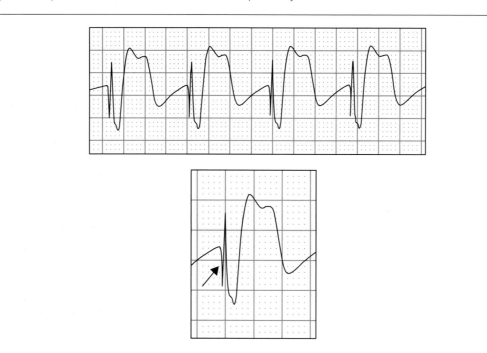

The QRS complex is widened due to impulse arrival at the ventricle within the ventricular myocardium without subsequent use of the His-Purkinje system for impulse conduction throughout the ventricle; the impulse is forced to move throughout the ventricular myocardium using myocyte-to-myocyte transmission—an inefficient means of impulse transmission, resulting in the widened QRS complex. Note the pacemaker spike (arrow), the narrow, vertically oriented line immediately preceding the QRS complex. Note that ST-segments cannot be interpreted accurately for acute myocardial ischemia in most instances.

14. **Sinus bradycardia (SB), rate 30, with frequent PVCs culminating in ventricular tachycardia, rate 180.** The underlying rhythm is SB. The rhythm is interrupted by wide QRS complex beats, that arrive early in the cycle—PVCs. The 3rd, 6th, and 7th beats in the top rhythm strip as well as the 2nd, 3rd, and 8th beats in the middle rhythm strip are PVCs. The first of the PVCs has a different morphology from the rest, indicating that it originates from a different ventricular focus. The bottom strip demonstrates a regular, wide QRS complex tachycardia. Normally the distinction between VT versus SVT with aberrant conduction is difficult in a single rhythm strip. In this case, however, VT is certain because the morphology of the QRS complexes in the tachycardic section is identical to the PVCs, indicating that they all are originating from the same ventricular focus.

15. **SR with second degree AV block type 2 (Mobitz II, high-grade AV block), rate 30.** P-waves appear regularly at a rate of 75 beats/minute. Multiple P-waves are non-conducted, however, indicating that either second or third degree AV block is present. Four QRS complexes appear, each preceded by the same PR-interval. This indicates that the QRS complexes are originating from the P-waves (ruling out AV dissociation and third degree AV block). Because the PR-intervals are constant in those P-waves that are conducted, second degree AV block type 2 (Mobitz II) is diagnosed. When Mobitz II exists and multiple consecutive P-waves are non-conducted, the rhythm is sometimes referred to as a "high-grade" AV block. The QRS complexes are wide, likely the result of some form of aberrant ventricular conduction.

16. **SR with second degree AV block type 2 (Mobitz II, high-grade AV block), rate 55, ST-segment depression consistent with cardiac ischemia.** Similar to the preceding case, there is evidence of regular atrial activity at a rate of 79 beats/minute and sequential P-waves in some areas are non-conducted. When P-waves *are* conducted, the PR-intervals remain constant. The diagnosis of Mobitz II conduction with high-grade AV block is made. The QRS complexes are wide suggesting aberrant ventricular conduction. Aberrant conduction is often associated with mild ST-segment elevation or depression in a direction that is opposite that of the main vector of the QRS complex (ST-segment "discordance"). However, when the discordance is >5 mm, as it is here, cardiac ischemia is usually present.

17. **Rhythm strip: ST, rate 140. ECG: ST, rate 180.** Both the rhythm strip and the ECG demonstrate regular, narrow QRS complex tachycardias. The differential diagnosis includes ST, SVT, and atrial flutter with 2:1 AV conduction. P-waves are noted preceding each QRS complex, consistent with ST. When rapid ventricular conduction is present, P-waves may be hidden, or "buried," within the T-waves and can be overlooked. A "camel-hump" morphology of the T-wave is often a clue to a buried P-wave, as seen in the rhythm strip as well as in lead II of the ECG.

18. **Rhythm strip: Paroxysmal supraventricular tachycardia, rate 265. ECG: Paroxysmal supraventricular tachycardia, rate 265.** As in the preceding case, a regular narrow QRS complex tachycardia is present. In contrast, however, ST is unlikely because neither the rhythm strip nor the ECG demonstrates obvious P-waves. Additionally, it would be unlikely even for an infant to mount a sinus tachycardia >220 beats/minute. Flutter waves are also absent, excluding the diagnosis of atrial flutter. The diagnosis of paroxysmal supraventricular tachycardia, or SVT, is made by exclusion. ST-segment depression is noted in multiple leads, a common finding in cases of SVT and without clinical relevance as long as the ST-segment depression resolves after conversion to SR.

19. This patient had a witnessed cardiac arrest and developed several rhythms during the course of his resuscitation.
    a) Ventricular fibrillation. The rhythm is chaotic without any obvious organized electrical activity. Ventricular fibrillation may be confused with artifact, but the two can be distinguished clinically—ventricular fibrillation does not produce a pulse. He is defibrillated to the rhythm in b).
    b) Probable accelerated idioventricular rhythm, rate 105. This is a fairly regular, wide QRS complex rhythm. Some atrial activity is noted but it is dissociated from the ventricular activity, suggesting that the QRS complexes

are originating in the ventricle. The rate is too fast to be defined as a simple ventricular escape rhythm (ventricular escape rhythms have a rate of 20–40 beats/minute), but not fast enough to be diagnosed as ventricular tachycardia (ventricular tachycardia requires a rate ≥120 beats/minute). When a ventricular rhythm is 40–120 beats/minute, the term *accelerated* ventricular rhythm, or accelerated idioventricular rhythm, is used. A pulse is noted.

c) ST, rate 160, ST-segment elevation (STE) consistent with acute MI. A regular, narrow QRS complex tachycardia is present with subtle P-waves preceding the QRS complexes. A slurred downstroke of the QRS complex appears, which likely represents the J-point (the point at which the QRS complex ends and the ST-segment begins), suggesting that STE is present.

d) ST, rate 115, STE consistent with acute MI. ST persists with STE, consistent with acute MI.

20. **Ventricular tachycardia (VT), rate 250.** Both the rhythm strip and the ECG demonstrate a regular, wide QRS complex tachycardia. The differential diagnosis includes VT, SVT with aberrant ventricular conduction, and ST with aberrant ventricular conduction. P-waves are occasionally noted but they are dissociated from the QRS complexes (AV dissociation), a finding that virtually confirms the diagnosis of VT.

21. **Accelerated junctional rhythm, rate 90, STE consistent with acute MI, PVCs with R-on-T phenomenon leading to polymorphic VT and ventricular fibrillation.** The initial portion of the rhythm is presumed to be an AV junctional rhythm because the QRS complexes are narrow and there are no preceding P-waves. Because the rate is faster than the intrinsic pacing rate of the AV junction (40–60 beats/minute), it is termed an accelerated junctional rhythm. The ST-segments appear to be elevated and convex upwards, consistent with an acute MI. A PVC appears on the terminal portion of the T-wave following the 6th QRS complex, precipitating a burst of polymorphic VT in the middle portion of the rhythm strip, and the rhythm then degenerates into the disorganized rhythm of ventricular fibrillation at the end of the rhythm strip. Premature ventricular depolarization during the ventricular repolarization phase can precipitate this type of rhythm degeneration and is referred to as "R-on-T phenomenon." See figure opposite.

22. **Atrial fibrillation, rate 140, aberrant ventricular conduction.** When the rhythm is irregularly irregular, the most common causes are atrial fibrillation, multifocal atrial tachycardia, and atrial flutter with variable AV conduction. Distinct P-waves or flutter waves are absent, excluding the latter two possibilities. The QRS complexes are wide, suggesting aberrant ventricular conduction. Aberrant conduction can be the result of a bundle branch block, metabolic abnormality (e.g. hyperkalemia), accessory pathway (e.g. WPW), or a non-specific intraventricular conduction delay. In the absence of a full 12-lead ECG, it is difficult to specify the exact cause of the aberrant conduction in this case.

23. **Multifocal atrial tachycardia (MAT), rate 130.** The rhythm is irregularly irregular. The differential diagnosis includes atrial fibrillation, MAT, and atrial flutter with variable conduction. In this case, P-waves are noted preceding the QRS complexes, and the P-waves have at least three distinct morphologies, indicating that they are originating from different foci within the atria. Thus, multifocal atrial tachycardia is diagnosed. This rhythm is most commonly encountered in patients with chronic pulmonary diseases.

24. **ST with AV dissociation and third degree AV block, AV junctional escape rhythm, rate 53.** P-waves are noted at a rate of 130 beats/minute. The QRS complexes are regular at a rate of 53 beats/minute. The atria and ventricles are beating at independent rates (AV dissociation) and there is no evidence that any of the P-waves are being conducted to the ventricles (third degree, or "complete," AV block). The QRS complexes are narrow and at a typical AV junctional rate (between 40–60 beats/minute), indicating that the escape rhythm is originating at the level of the AV junction.

This figure corresponds to case #21

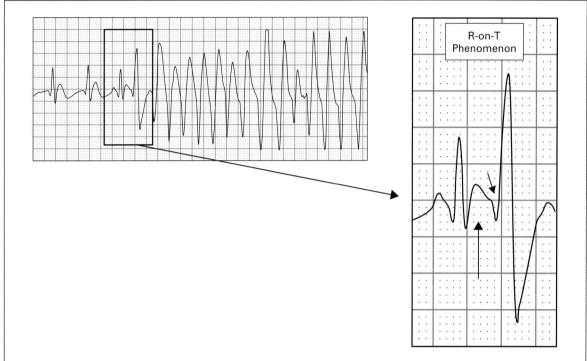

The R-on-T phenomenon describes the delivery of an electrical discharge (R-wave denoted by small arrow) on an electrically vulnerable period of the electrocardiographic cycle (T-wave as denoted by large arrow). Subsequent to this PVC, coarse ventricular fibrillation results.

25. **Polymorphic VT, suspected torsade de pointes, rate 350.** The initial QRS complex appears to be a sinus beat, which is then followed by R-on-T phenomenon (see case #21) producing polymorphic VT. The QRS complexes appear to rotate around a fixed point, growing larger, then smaller, then larger, and so on. This pattern is suggestive of torsade de pointes (see case #3). Confirmation of torsades de pointes would require the finding of a prolonged QT-interval during sinus rhythm either before initiation of the polymorphic VT or after conversion.

Reference
1.   Priori SG, Schwartz PJ, Napolitano C, *et al.* Risk stratification in the long-QT syndrome. *N Engl J Med* 2003;**348**:1866–74.

Part 2
12-Lead ECGs (intermediate level)

Case histories

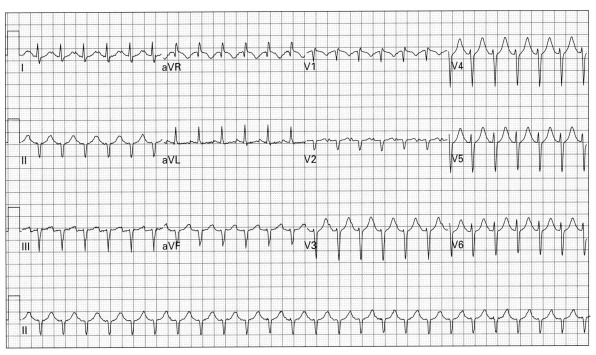

26. 56 year old man presents with fever, tachypnea, and hypotension

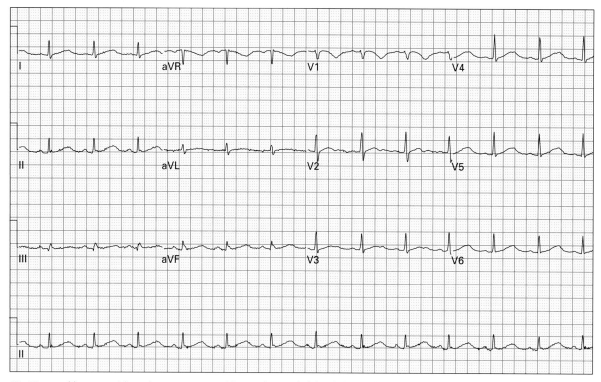

27. 51 year old woman with persistent nausea, vomiting, and severe lightheadedness after attending a picnic

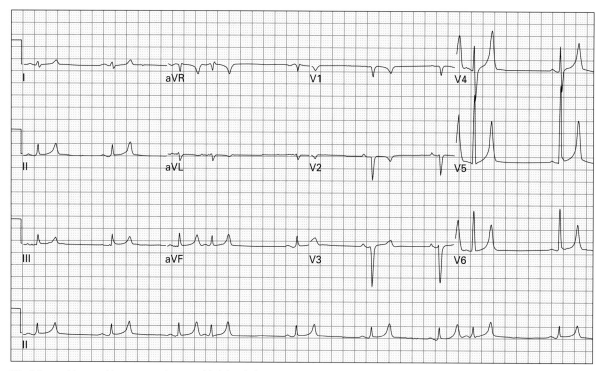

28. 26 year old man with severe weakness and lightheadedness

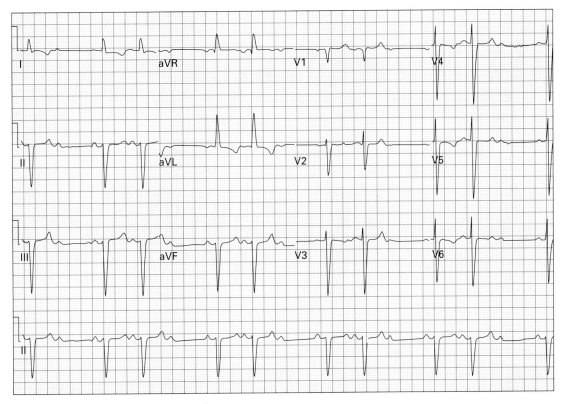

29. 55 year old man presents after syncopal episode

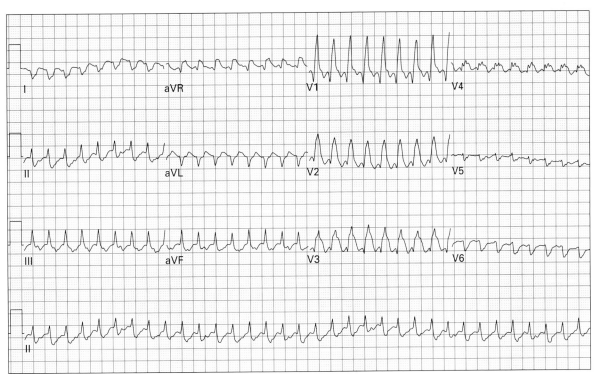

30. 45 year old man with palpitations and lightheadedness

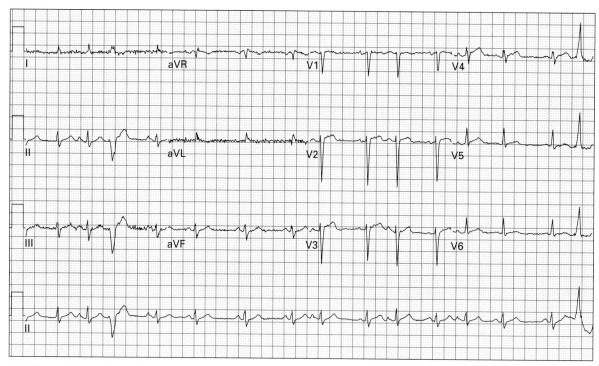

31. 72 year old man with emphysema presents with dyspnea

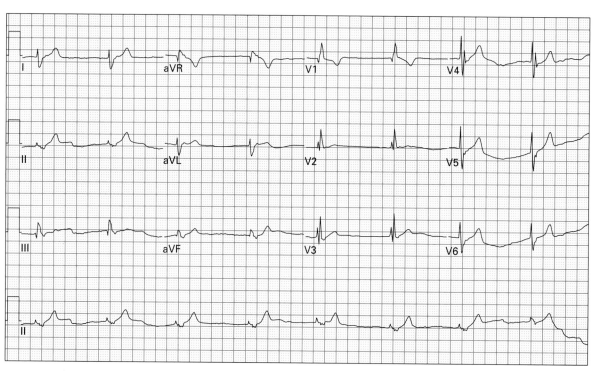

32. 49 year old man with severe lightheadedness

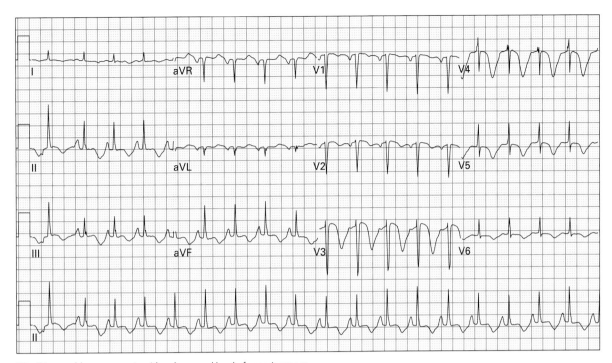

33. 61 year old man presents with a decreased level of consciousness

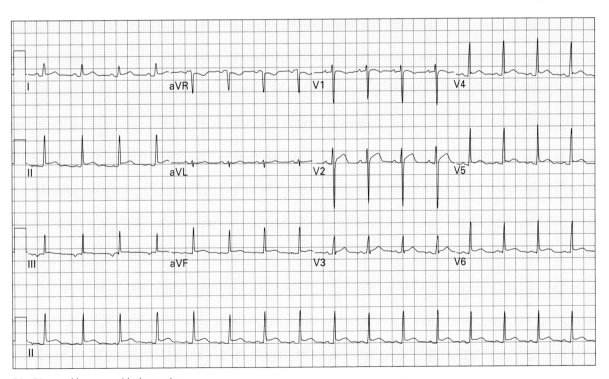

34. 21 year old woman with chest pain

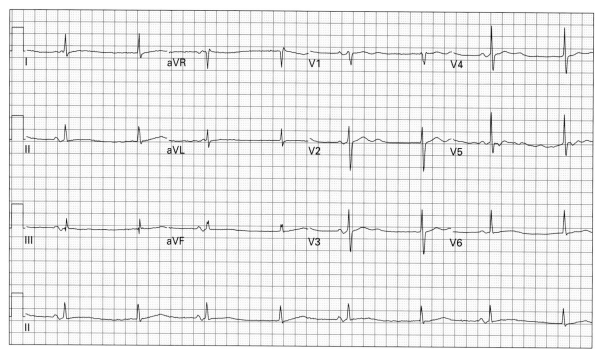

35. 69 year old man with lightheadedness after starting new medications

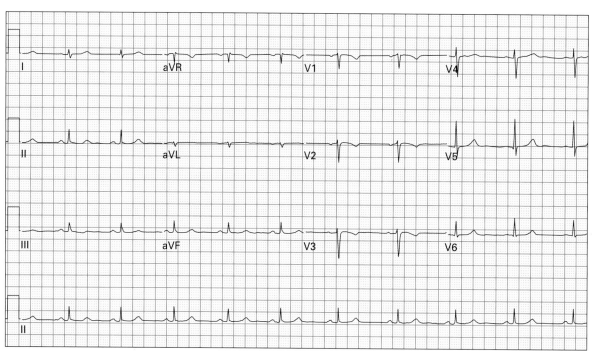

36. 38 year old woman with atypical chest pain

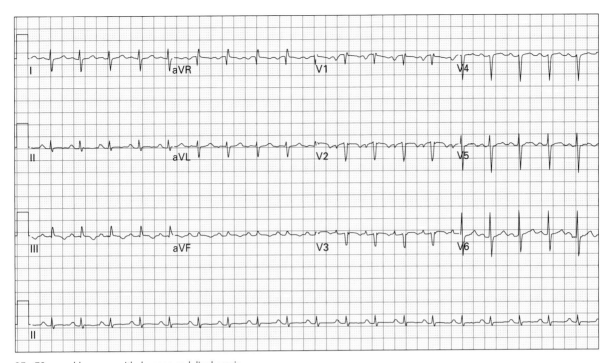

37. 72 year old woman with dyspnea and diaphoresis

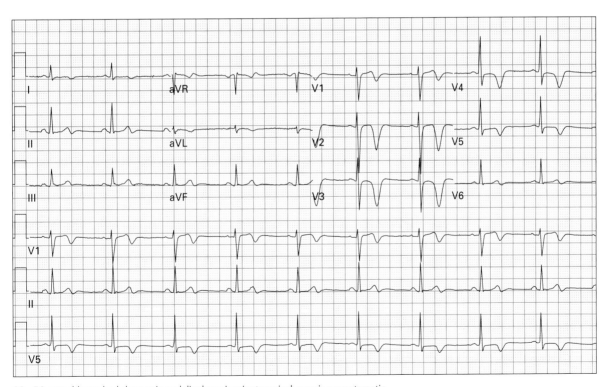

38. 56 year old man had chest pain and diaphoresis prior to arrival, now is asymptomatic

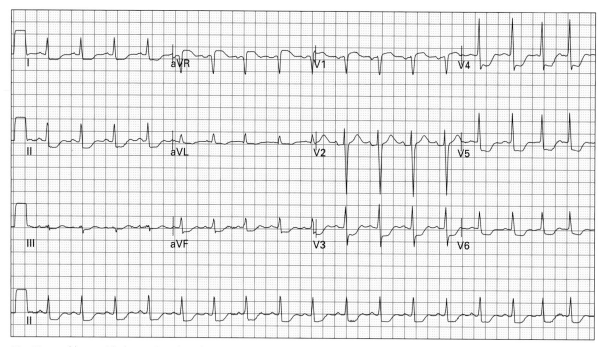

39. 68 year old man with chest pain and weakness

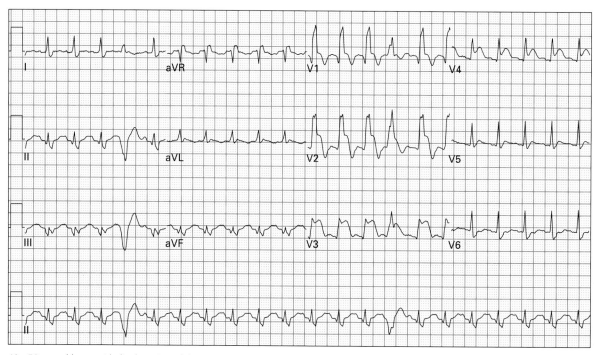

40. 58 year old man with diaphoresis and dyspnea

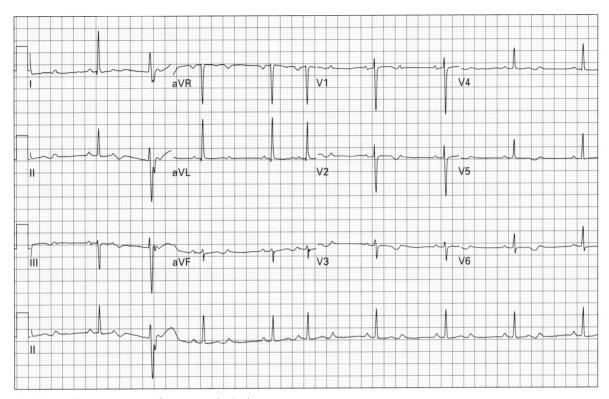

41. 76 year old woman presents after a syncopal episode

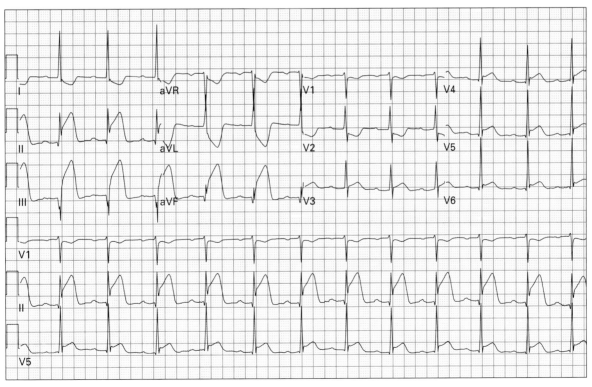

42. 46 year old man with chest pressure and lightheadedness

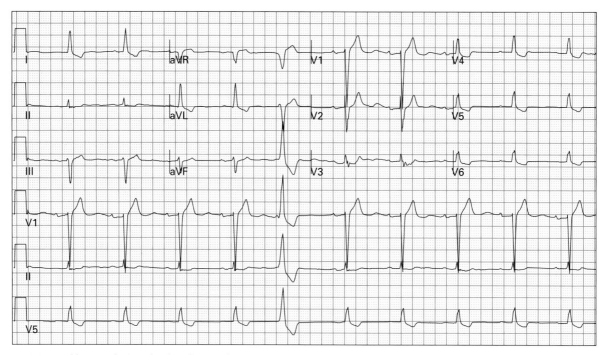

43. 85 year old man with generalized weakness and nausea

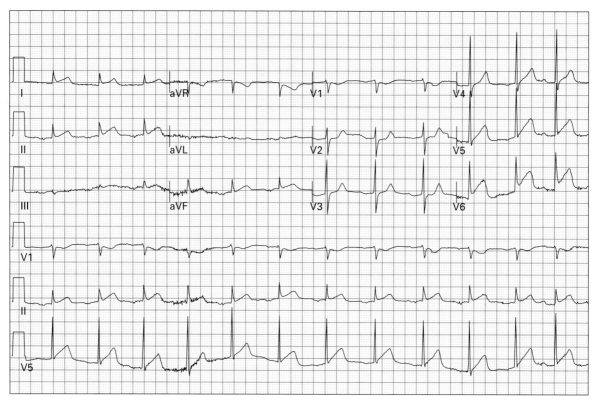

44. 82 year old man with severe weakness and diaphoresis

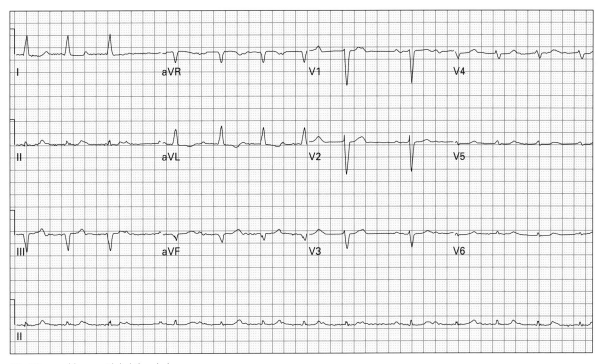

45. 75 year old man with lightheadedness

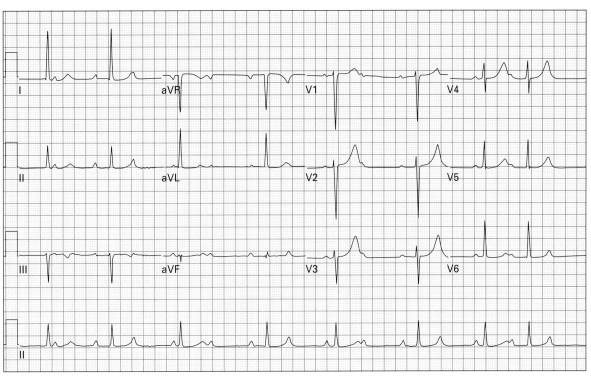

46. 37 year old man with diffuse myalgias, severe weakness, and a large rash on his torso

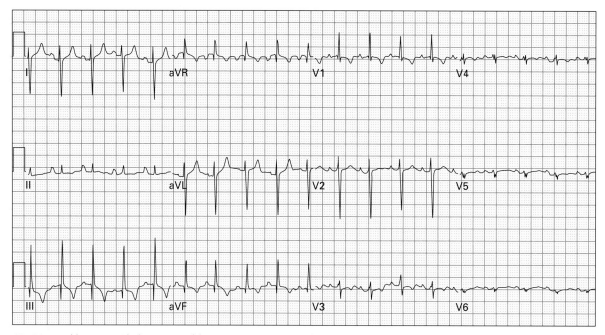

47. 54 year old woman with chest pain and dyspnea

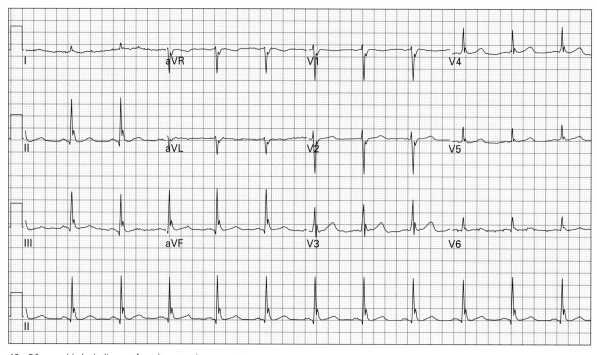

48. 56 year old alcoholic man found unconscious

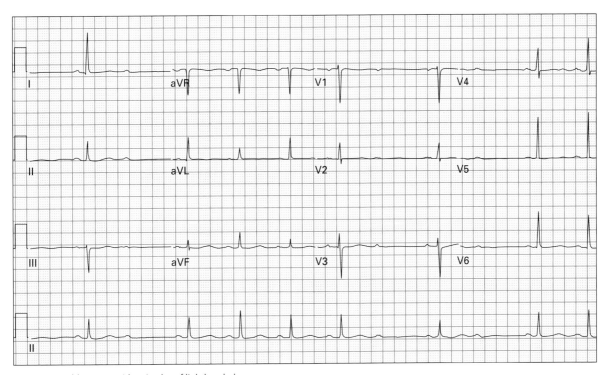

49. 74 year old woman with episodes of lightheadedness

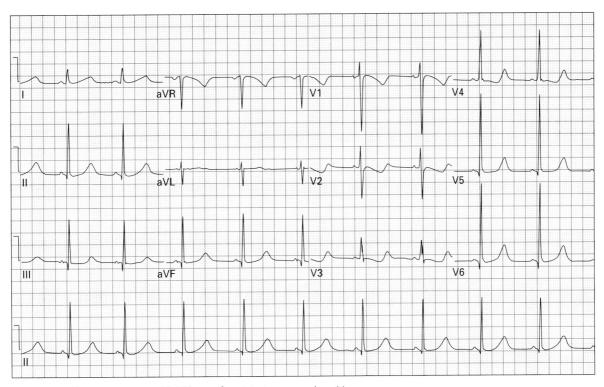

50. 20 year old pregnant woman with 12 hours of persistent nausea and vomiting

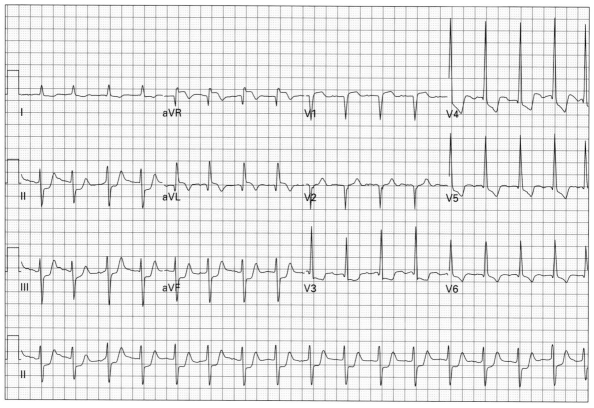

51. 84 year old man had syncopal episode while driving, no injuries

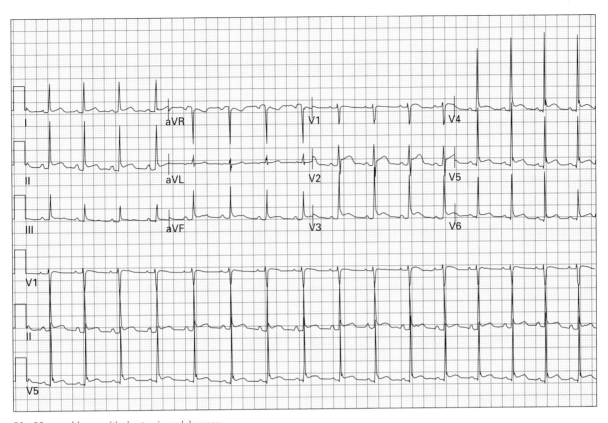

52. 29 year old man with chest pain and dysnpea

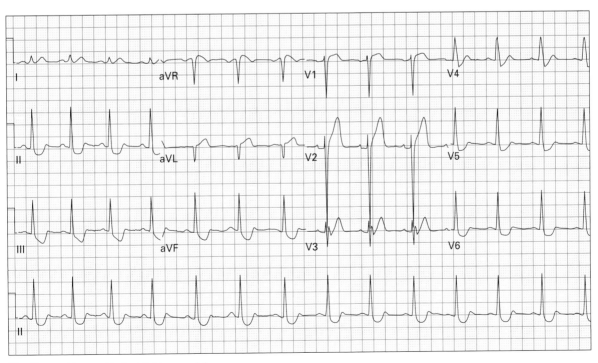

53. 28 year old man with chest tightness and dyspnea

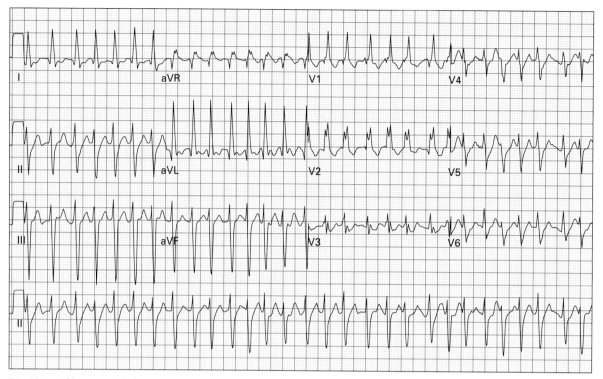

54. 83 year old woman with dyspnea

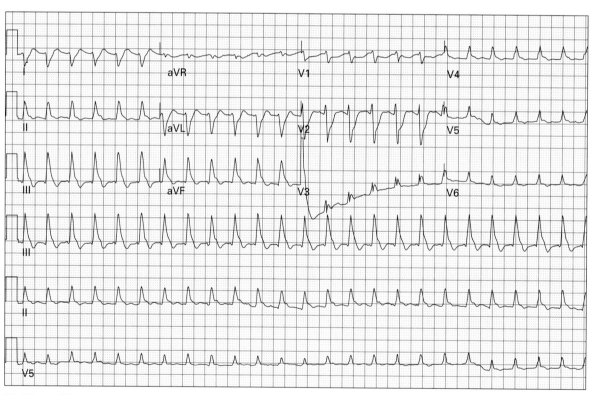

55. 75 year old woman presents unconsciousness after resuscitation from cardiac arrest

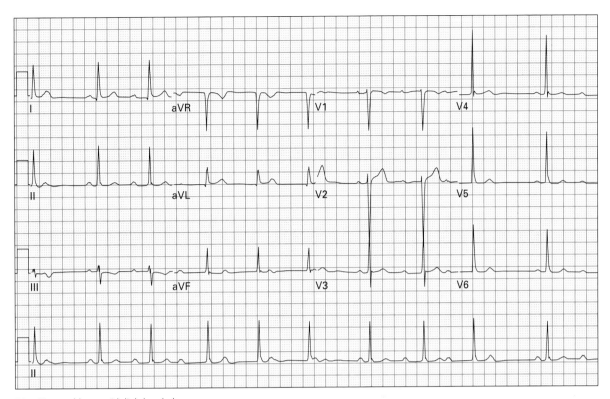

56. 45 year old man with lightheadedness

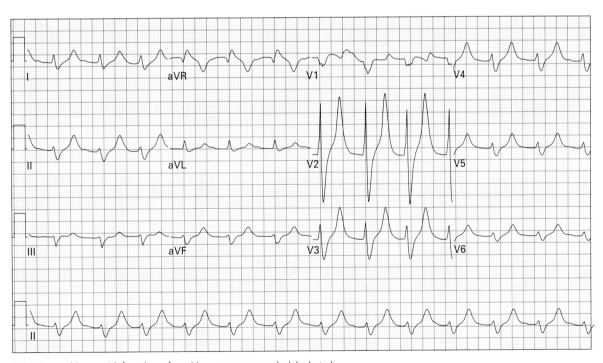

57. 70 year old man with four days of vomiting, appears severely dehydrated

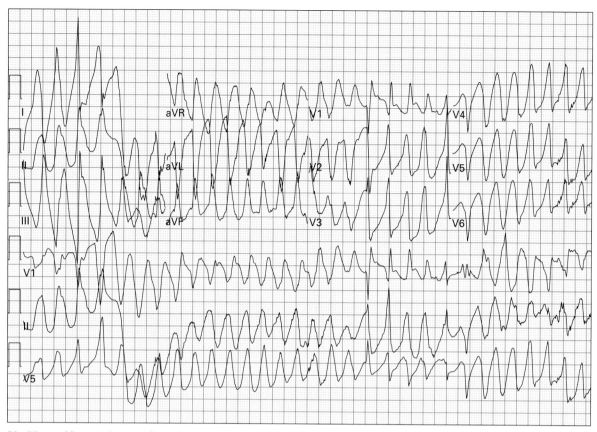

58. 55 year old man with syncopal episodes

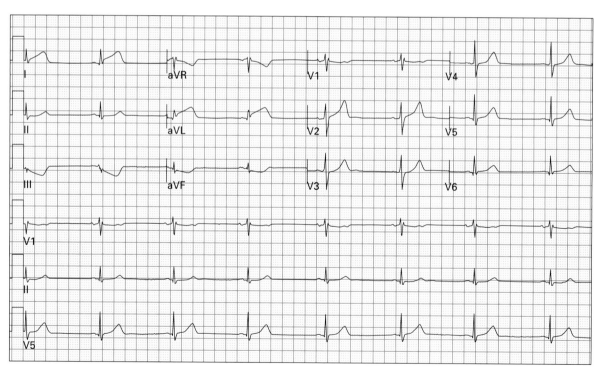

59. 60 year old man with chest pressure and diaphoresis

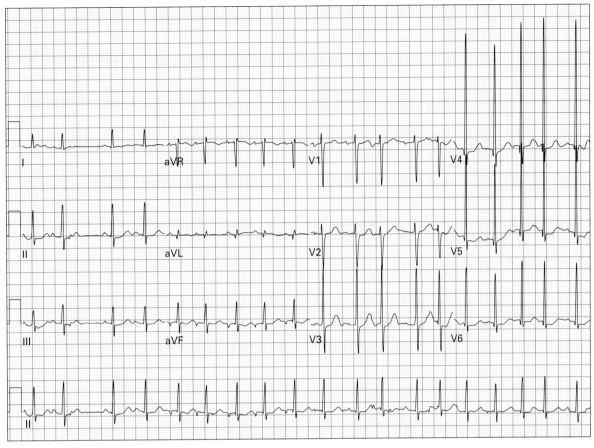

60. 61 year old woman with dyspnea and hypoxia

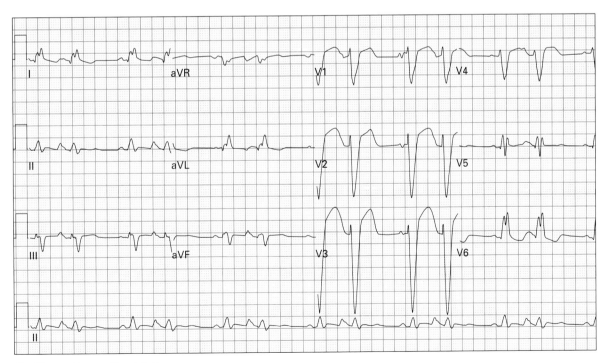

61. 65 year old man with palpitations

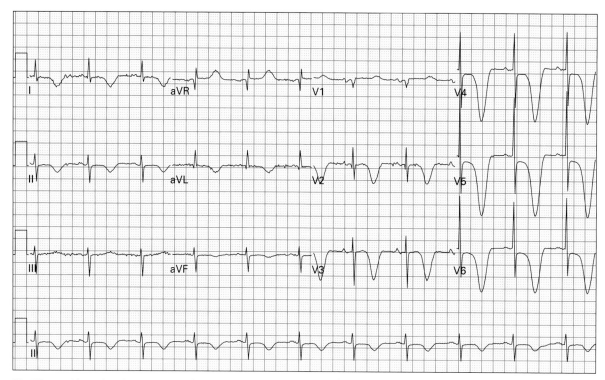

62. 77 year old man found unconscious at home

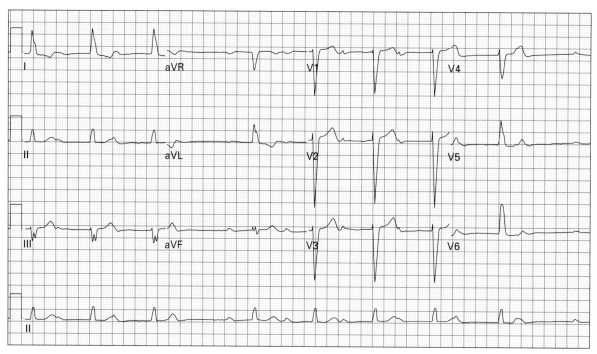

63. 93 year old woman presents after a syncopal episode

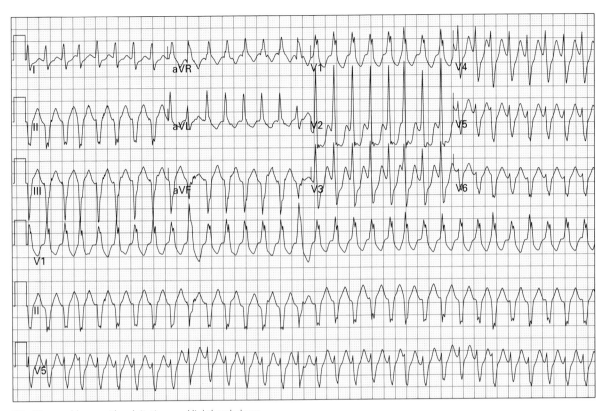

64. 55 year old man with palpitations and lightheadedness

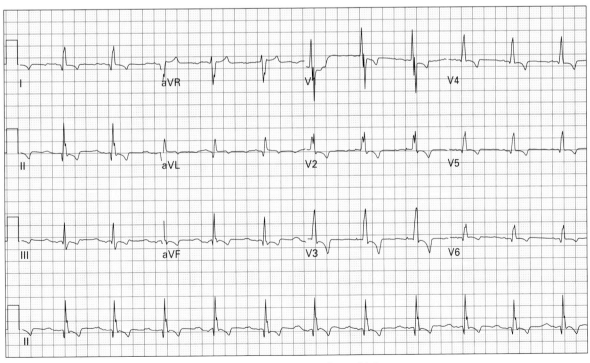

65. 59 year old man with dyspnea after missing his last hemodialysis session for renal failure

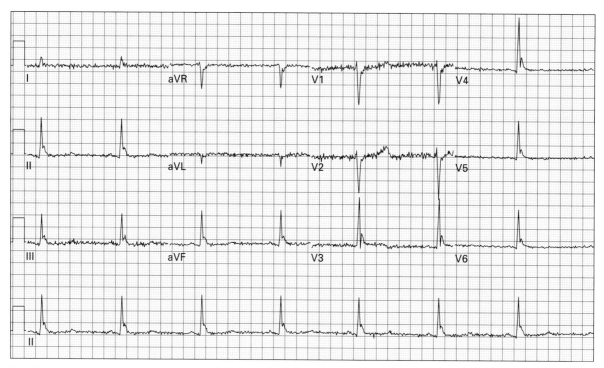

66. 49 year old alcoholic man found unconscious lying in an alley

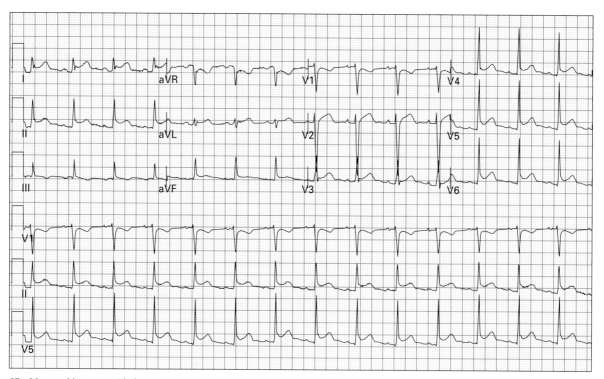

67. 32 year old woman with dyspnea

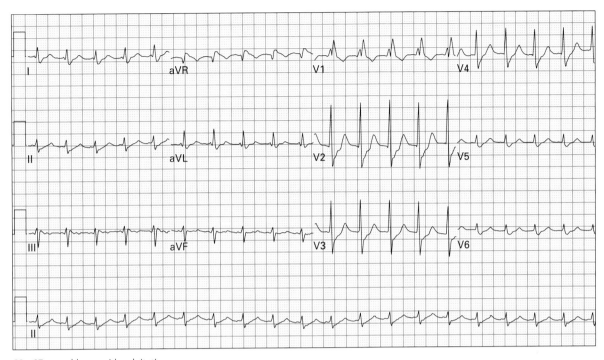

68. 67 year old man with palpitations

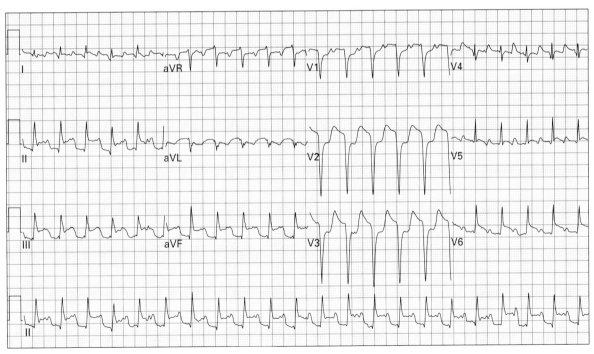

69. 53 year old man with prior history of MI presents with chest pain and diaphoresis

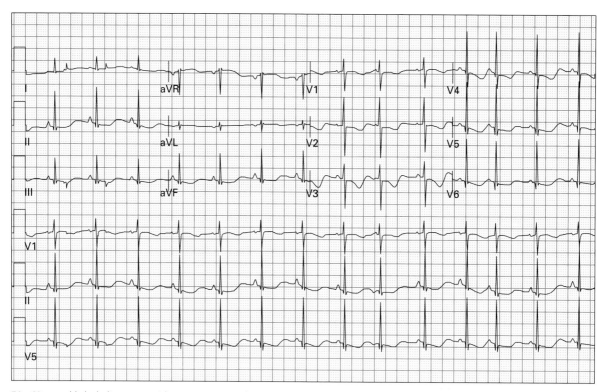

70. 63 year old alcoholic woman with severe nausea and vomiting

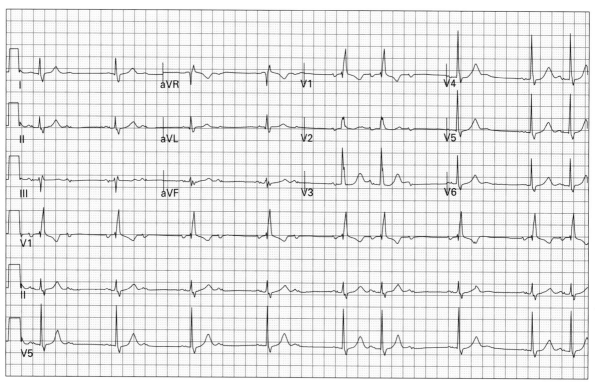

71. 74 year old man presents after a syncopal episode

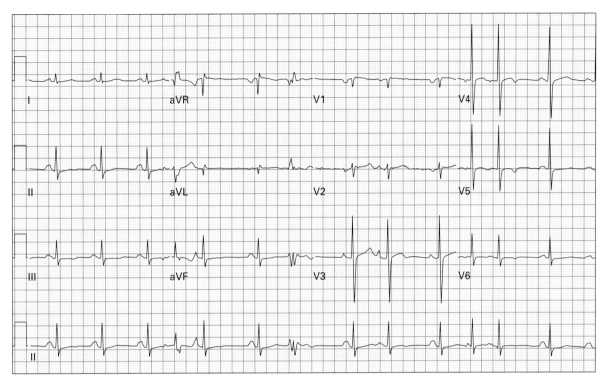

72. 53 year old man with an acute asthma exacerbation

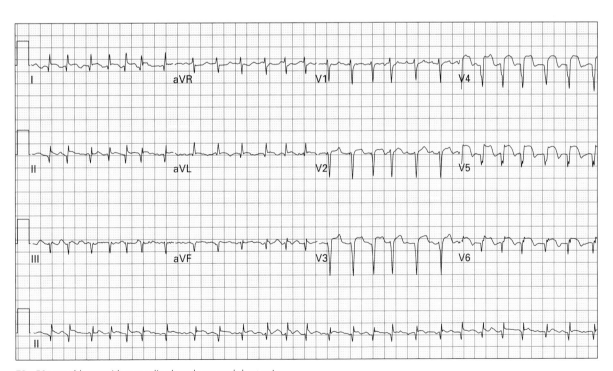

73. 59 year old man with generalized weakness and chest pain

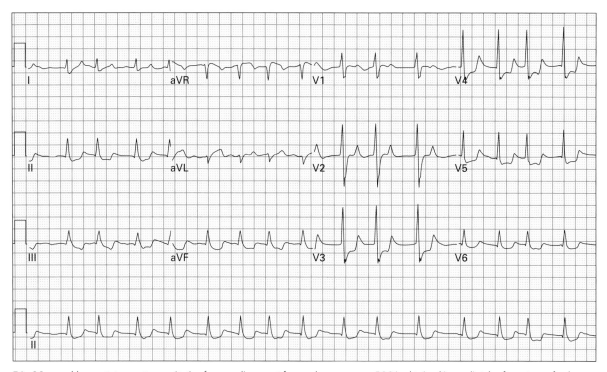

74. 36 year old man status post resuscitation from cardiac arrest from unknown cause; ECG is obtained immediately after return of pulses

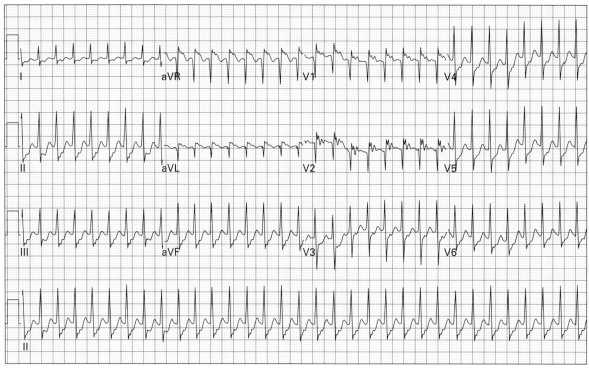

75. 60 year old woman with palpitations while receiving continues beta-agonist nebulizers for asthma

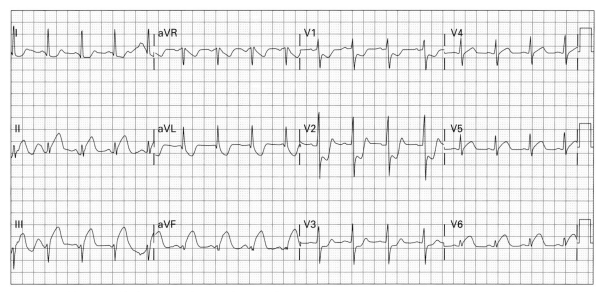

76. 46 year old woman with chest pain and acute pulmonary edema

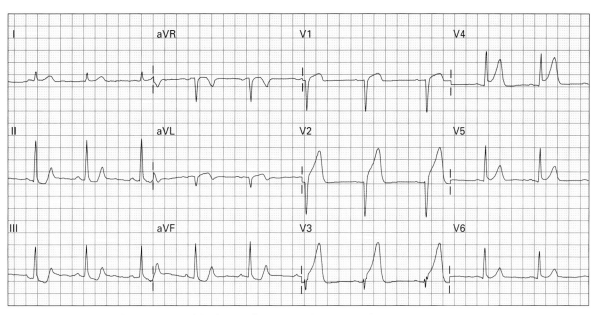

77. 41 year old man with chest pressure and diaphoresis of approximately 30 minutes duration

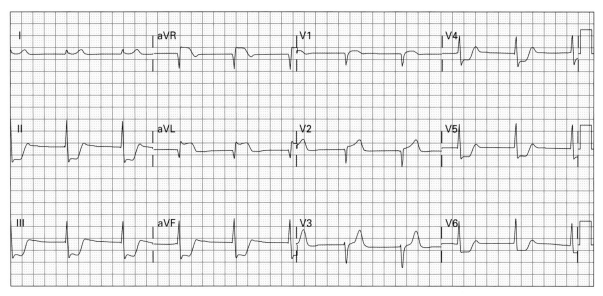

78. 53 year old man with chest pain and hypotension

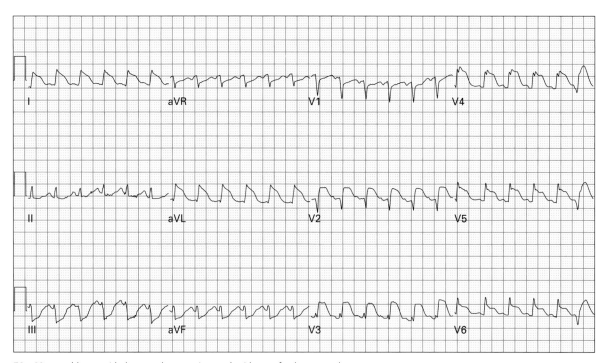

79. 68 year old man with dyspnea, hypotension, and evidence of pulmonary edema

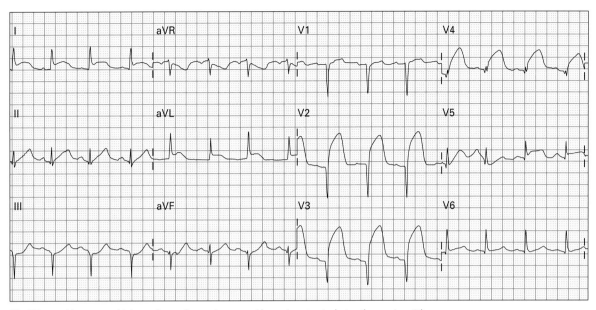

80. 57 year old woman with intermittent chest pain, now with persistent pain during the previous 3 hours

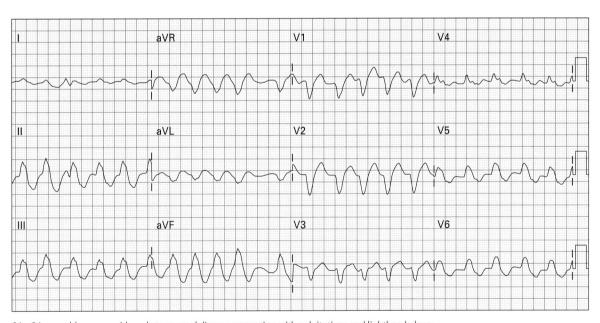

81. 31 year old woman with end-stage renal disease presenting with palpitations and lightheadedness

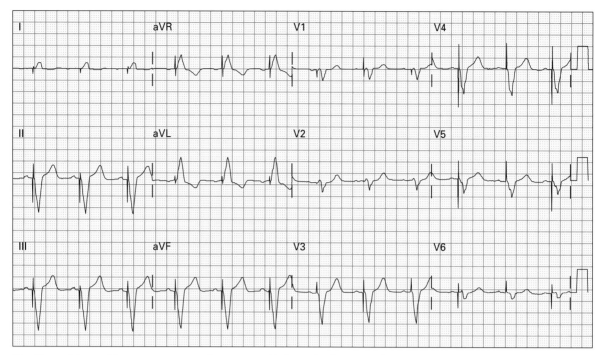

82. 62 year old man with a permanent pacemaker presents with chest pain, dyspnea, and nausea

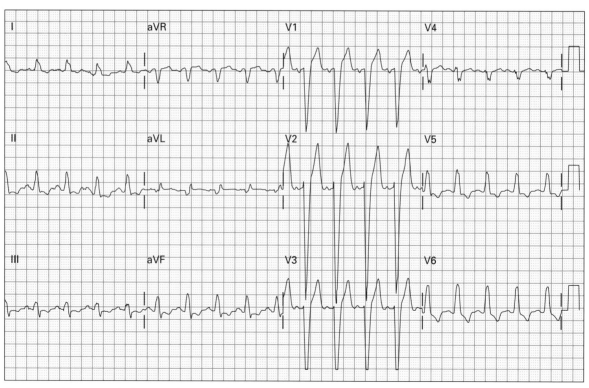

83. 54 year old woman with chest pain, dyspnea, and diaphoresis

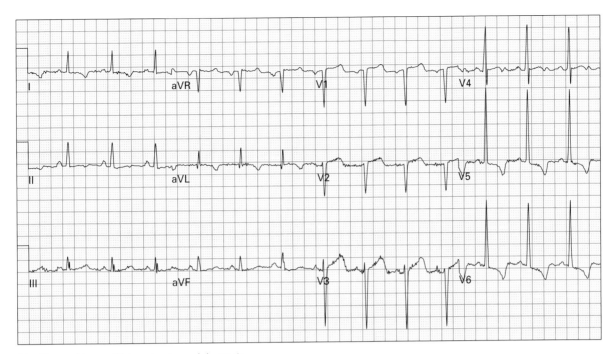

84. 60 year old man with hypertension and chest pain

a)

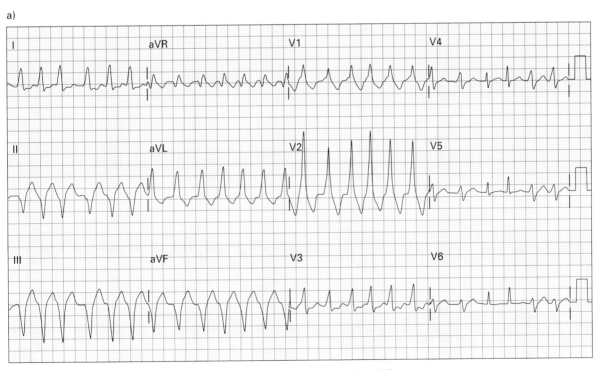

85. 21 year old woman with palpitations and dizziness, a) upon arrival, (*continued on p. 60*)

b)

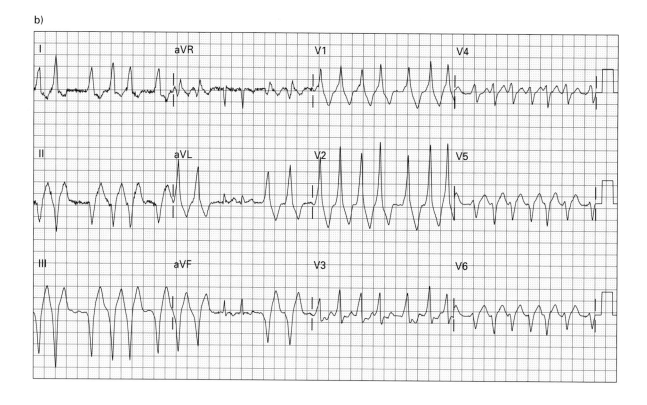

c)

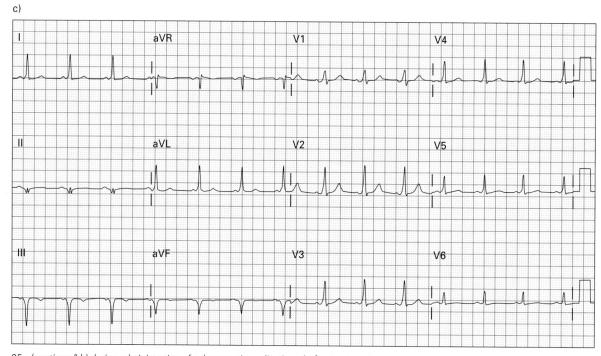

85. (*continued*) b) during administration of a therapeutic medication, c) after treatment

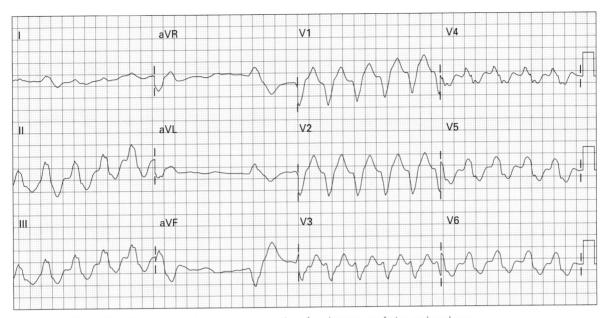

86. 12 year old boy with failed renal transplant who presents with profound nausea, confusion, and weakness

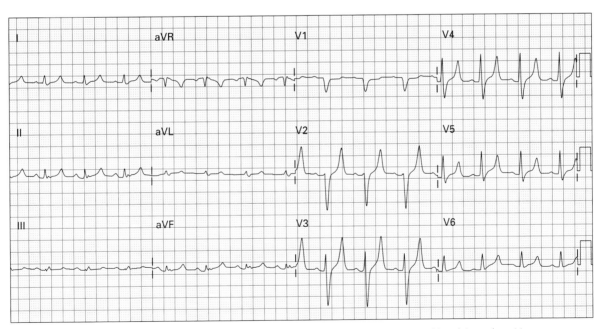

87. 39 year old man with alcoholic liver disease managed with potassium-sparing diuretic presents with malaise and vomiting

a)

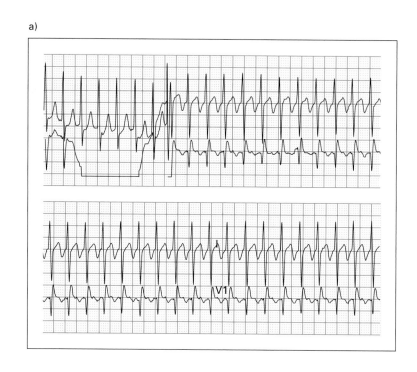

b)

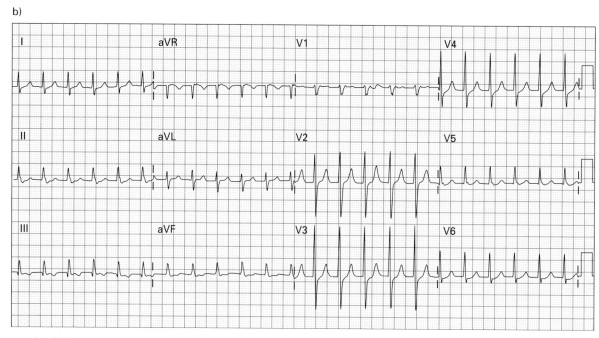

88. a) and b) 69 year old woman with weakness and palpitations

a)

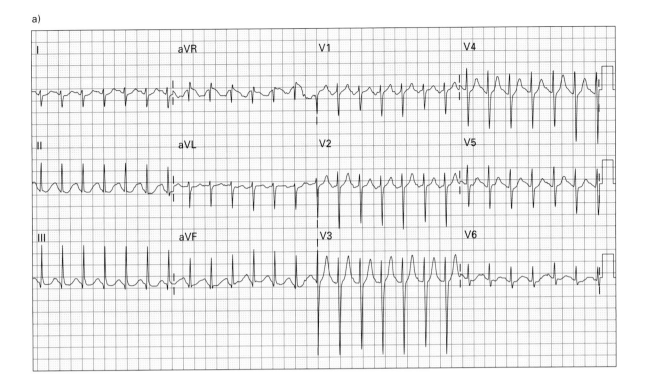

b)

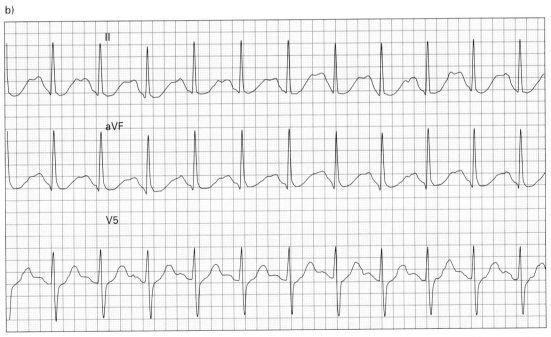

89. 38 year old woman with theophylline overdose, a) standard 12-lead ECG, b) rhythm strip at rapid chart speed (50 mm/sec)

a)

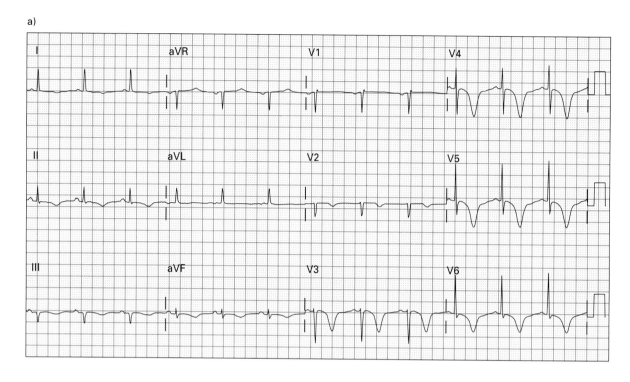

b)

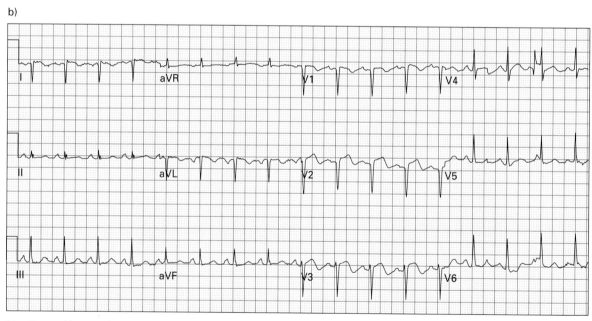

90. 45 year old man with recent chest pain who presents now pain-free, a) initial ECG, b) 2 days later

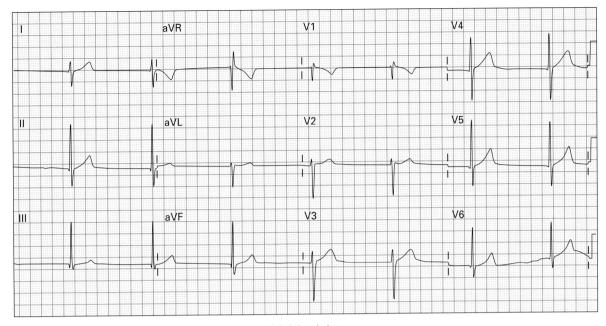

91. 67 year old woman with sick sinus syndrome presents with lightheadedness

a)

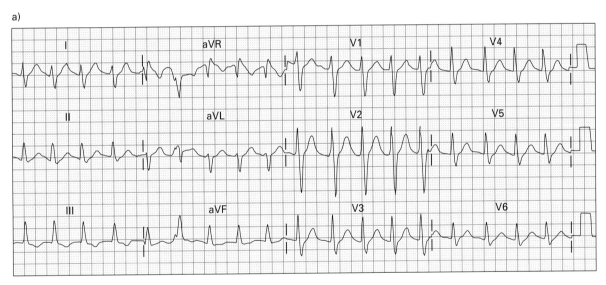

b)

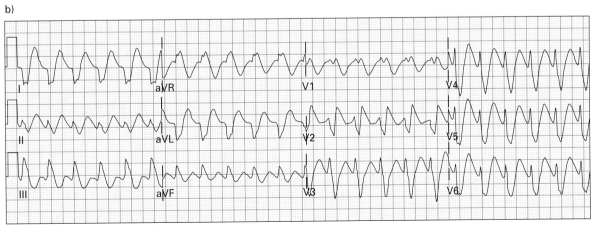

92. 29 year old woman with recent overdose of her "nerve pill", a) initial ECG, b) without therapy, 30 minutes later

a)

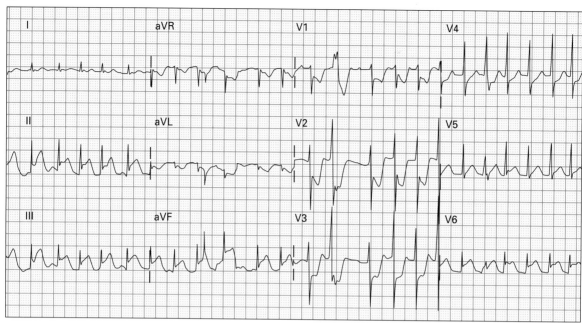

b)

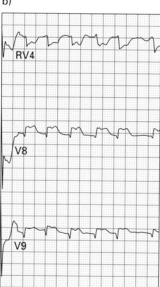

93. 41 year old man with chest pain, a) initial ECG, b) right-side (RV4) and posterior-placed (V8, V9) leads

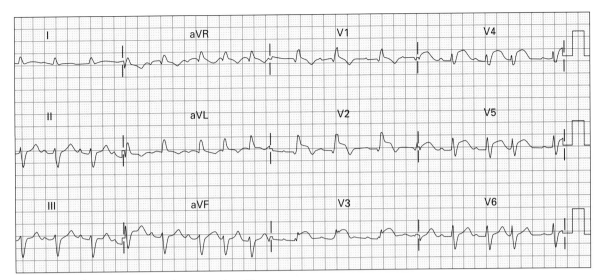

94. 58 year old with chest pressure, dyspnea, and vomiting

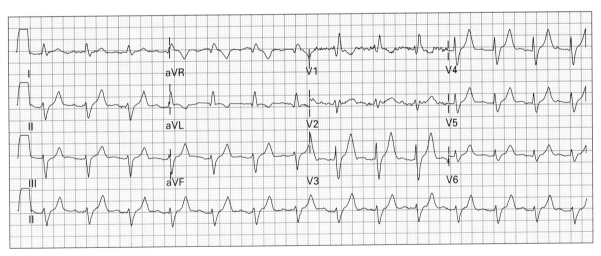

95. 56 year old man with diarrhea and profound dehydration

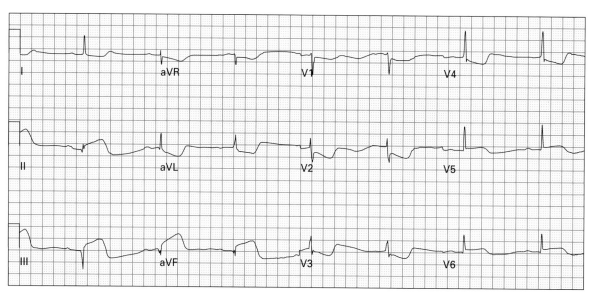

96. 40 year old man with chest pain and hypotension

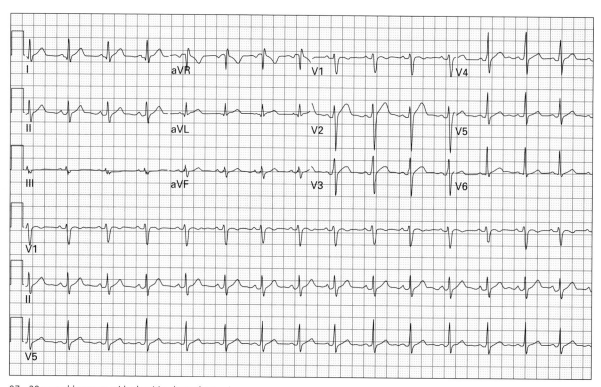

97. 29 year old woman with pleuritic, sharp chest pain

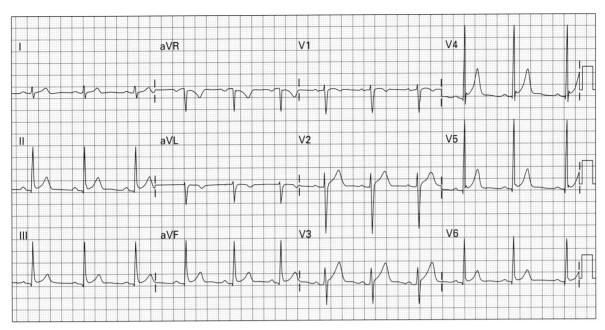

98. 31 year old woman with chest pain after cocaine use

a)

b)

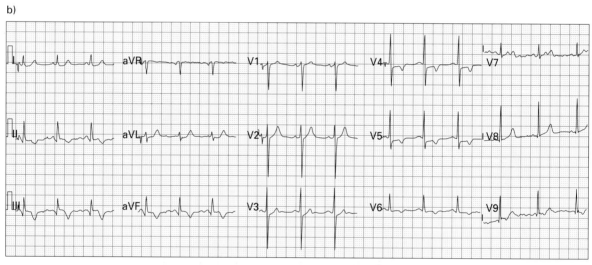

99. 54 year old woman with chest pain, a) initial ECG, b) 15-lead ECG, (*continued opposite*)

c)

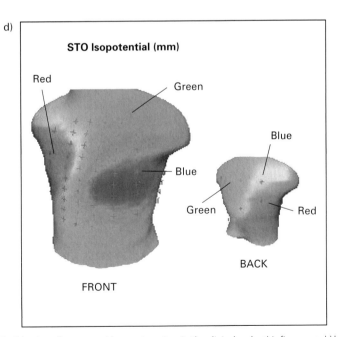

d)

STO Isopotential (mm)

FRONT

BACK

99. (*continued*) c) 80-lead ECG, d) body surface map with torso imaging. In the clinical realm this figure would be depicted in colour. Red represents ST segment elevation, blue represents ST segment depression, green represents normal-ST segment.

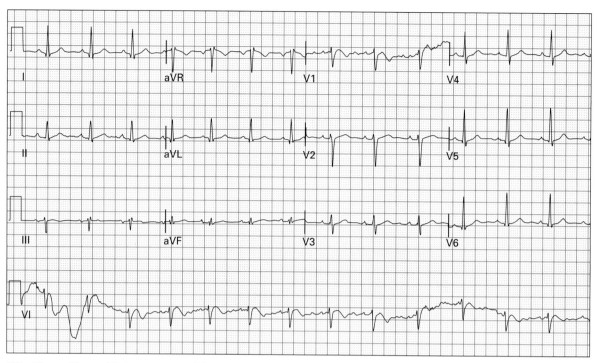

100. 46 year old man with chest pressure and dyspnea

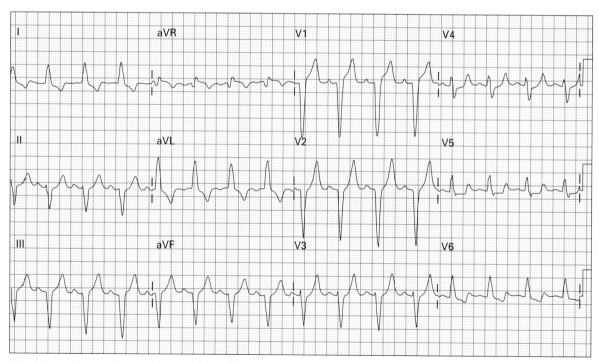

101. 79 year old man with acute dyspnea and chest tightness

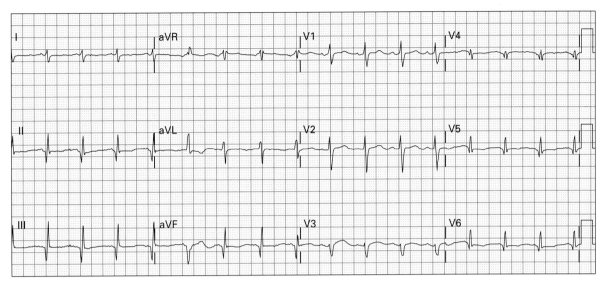

102. 67 year old patient with a history of past myocardial infarction and gastroesophageal reflux presents with belching and substernal burning sensation

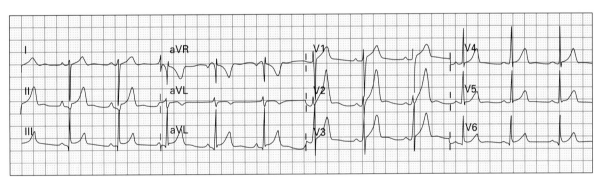

103. 32 year old man with recent cocaine use and chest pain

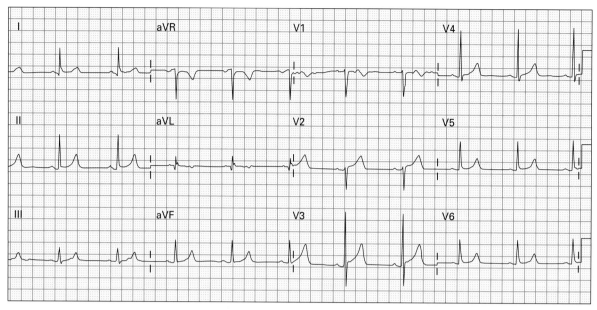

104. 29 year old man with sharp chest pain

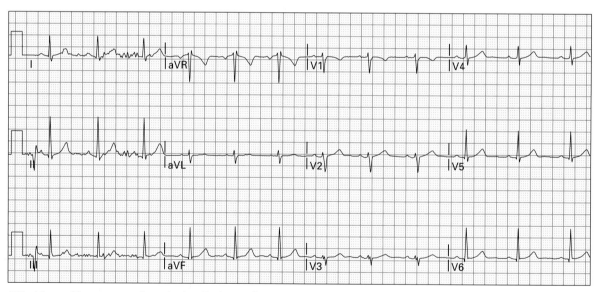

105. 17 year old man presents for evaluation 45 minutes after an intentional ingestion of a relative's medications (psychiatric and cardiovascular)

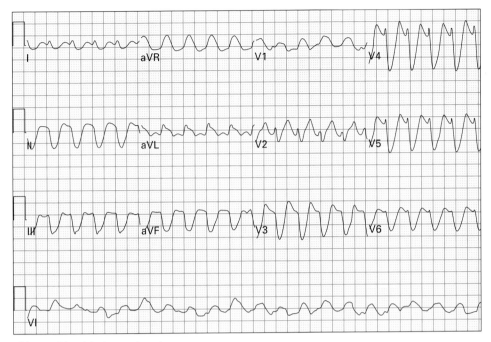

106. 45 year old man with palpitations and weakness

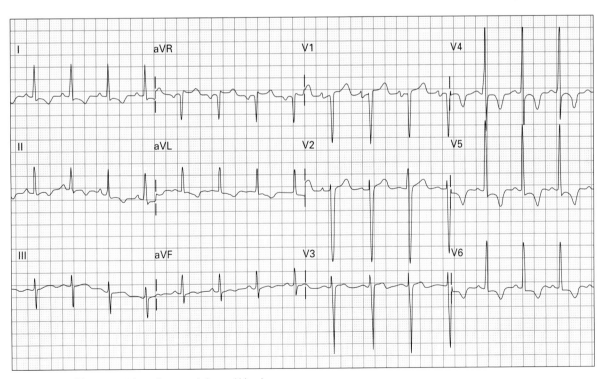

107. 59 year old woman with weakness and elevated blood pressure

a)

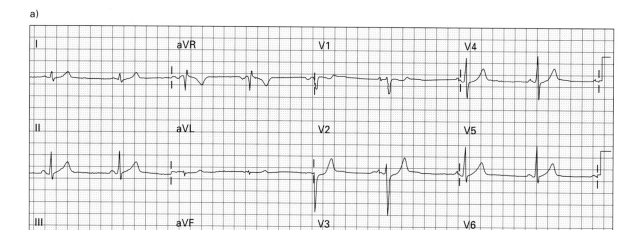

b)

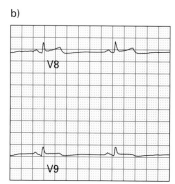

108. 49 year old man with substernal chest pressure, a) 12-lead ECG, b) posterior leads V8 and V9

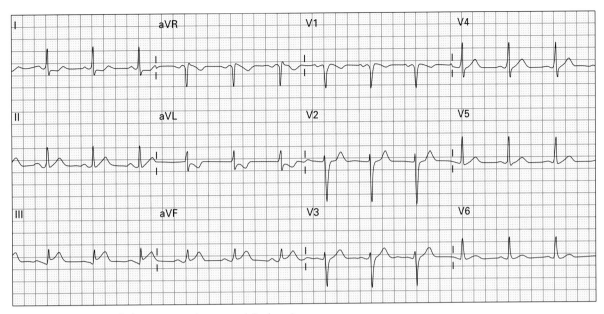

109. 56 year old man with chest pressure, dyspnea, and diaphoresis

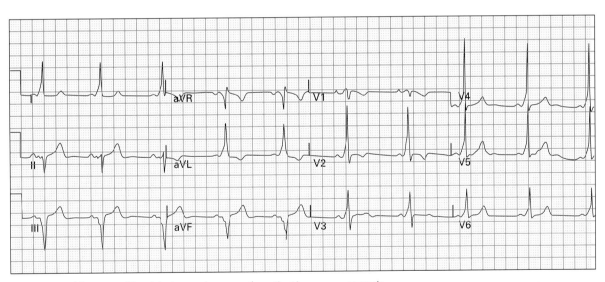

110. 16 year old woman with palpitations and syncope; the patient is now asymptomatic

ECG interpretations
and comments

(Rates refer to ventricular rate unless otherwise indicated)

26. **Sinus tachycardia (ST), rate 150, left anterior fascicular block (LAFB), septal infarct of undetermined age.** The patient presents with a narrow-complex, regular tachycardia. The differential diagnosis of narrow regular tachycardias primarily consists of only three entities: sinus tachycardia, supraventricular tachycardia (SVT), and atrial flutter (with 2:1 atrio-ventricular conduction). P-waves are best seen preceding the QRS complexes in lead V2, and they also appear more subtly embedded in the terminal portion of the T-waves in leads I and V3. The regular P-QRS association rules out SVT, and the lack of flutter waves rules out atrial flutter. LAFB is diagnosed based on the presence of a leftward axis, the presence of rS complexes in lead III, and qR complexes in leads I and aVL. Q waves are noted in leads V1 and V2 without ST or T-wave abnormalities, indicative of prior septal infarction. This patient was determined to have severe sepsis, the cause of tachycardia. The initial ECG interpretation was SVT because the rhythm diagnosis was based only on inspection of lead II. In this ECG, P-waves are not well seen in lead II.

27. **Sinus rhythm (SR), rate 82, prolonged QT-interval, U-waves suggestive of hypokalemia.** SR is generally defined as having an atrial rate of 60–100/minute and a P-wave axis of +15 to +75 degrees. Sinus beats can be defined by upright P-waves in leads I, II, III, and aVF, and inverted P-waves in lead aVR. The QT-interval varies based on the rate. The Bazett formula provides a correction factor based on the rate, whereby the corrected QT (QTc) = $QT/\sqrt{(RR)}$. QTc is considered prolonged when >450 msec in men and >460 msec in women and children. Causes of prolonged QTc include hypokalemia, hypomagnesemia, hypocalcemia, acute myocardial ischemia, elevated intracranial pressure, drugs with sodium channel blocking effects, hypothermia, and congenital prolonged QT syndrome. Patients with prolonged QTc, especially >500 msec, are at risk for developing torsades de pointes (TDP). The QTc in this ECG is 650 msec. Small U-waves are noted in leads V2–V3. Ordinarily these might be considered non-specific; however, in the presence of the prolonged QTc, they are suggestive of hypokalemia.

    While awaiting laboratory studies, the patient developed TDP but was quickly resuscitated. It was later discovered that the serum potassium level was 2.9 mEq/L (normal 3.5–5.3 mEq/L) and the serum magnesium level was 1.2 mEq/L (normal 1.4–2.0 mEq/L). Correction of the electrolyte abnormalities resulted in normalization of the QTc.

28. **Sinus bradycardia (SB), rate 45, frequent premature atrial complexes (PACs) in a pattern of quadrigeminy, peaked T-waves suggestive of hyperkalemia.** The overall rhythm is regularly irregular. Regular irregularity should suggest one of two possibilities: second degree atrioventricular (AV) block or regular-occurring PACs. Second degree AV block is ruled out because all of the P-waves are conducted. On the other hand, PACs appear every fourth beat and are followed by a pause in the regular cycle of beats. Peaked T-waves are noted in the lateral precordial leads as well, diagnostic of hyperkalemia. Hyperkalemia-associated T-waves can be distinguished from other causes of large T-waves by their narrow base, symmetric shape, and "sharp," peaked apex. Other causes of large T-waves tend to be more broad-based and more rounded at the apex. The serum potassium level was 8.3 mEq/L. Although common teaching regarding ECG manifestations of hyperkalemia focuses on peaked T-waves, widening of the QRS complex, and ventricular dysrhythmias; hyperkalemia is well-known to produce unusual bradycardias, AV blocks, fascicular blocks, and bundle branch blocks as well.

29. **SR with second degree AV block type 2 (Mobitz II), rate 60, left ventricular hypertrophy with repolarization abnormality and QRS widening.** SR is diagnosed based on upright P-waves in leads I, II, III, and aVF with inverted P-waves in aVR. The atrial rate is approximately 90/minute. Mobitz II AV conduction is diagnosed here based on the following: (1) presence of regular atrial activity (P-waves are regular), (2) some P-waves are non-conducted, and (3) in all of the conducted beats, the PR interval remains constant. The conduction of the P-waves occurs in a regular 3:2 ratio (3 P-waves for every 2 QRS complexes). Left ventricular hypertrophy (LVH) is diagnosed based on the R-wave amplitude in aVL >11 mm. LVH is often associated with abnormal repolarization, manifest as inverted T-waves in the lateral leads (I, aVL, V4–V6) and slight prolongation of the QRS complex. Leftward axis is noted as well. Causes of leftward axis include LVH, left bundle branch block (LBBB), prior inferior wall MI, left anterior fascicular block (LAFB), ventricular ectopy, paced beats, and Wolff-Parkinson-White syndrome. The leftward axis noted in this ECG is related to LVH. See figure below.

This figure corresponds to case #29. Second degree AV block type 2 is an advanced form of AV conduction abnormality with significant risk to the patient

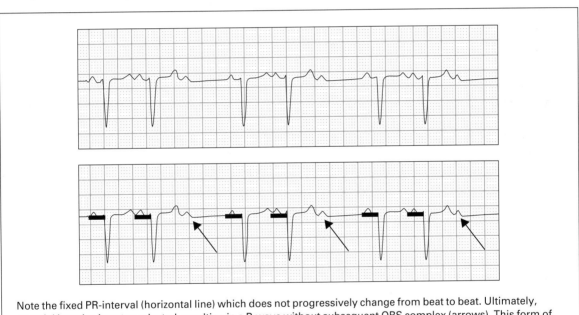

Note the fixed PR-interval (horizontal line) which does not progressively change from beat to beat. Ultimately, an atrial impulse is not conducted, resulting in a P-wave without subsequent QRS complex (arrows). This form of AV block should be considered malignant, with concern for progression to third degree (complete) heart block.

30. **Ventricular tachycardia, rate 205.** The ECG demonstrates a regular wide-QRS complex tachycardia (WCT). The primary considerations with a regular WCT are ventricular tachycardia (VT), supraventricular tachycardia (SVT) with aberrant conduction, and ST with aberrant conduction. ST can be excluded by the absence of regular sinus P-waves. Additionally, the rate of 205 is too fast for sinus activity—the maximal sinus rate of a patient can be estimated by 220 – age, which in this patient would be 175/minute. In deciding between VT versus SVT with aberrant conduction, WCTs should almost always be assumed to represent ventricular tachycardia, even in patients such as this one who are relatively young. In this case, ECG findings that further confirm the presence of VT are rightward axis, which is rare in cases of SVT with aberrant conduction, and the presence of AV dissociation, which confirms VT. See figure on p. 80.

This figure corresponds to case #30

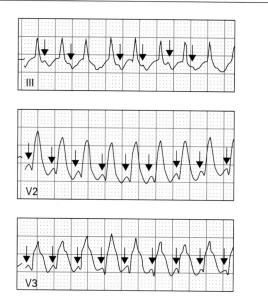

Accurate interpretation of wide QRS complex tachycardias can be a significant challenge. One of the electrocardiographic features which can assist the clinician with the evaluation of the dysrhythmia and aid in the ECG diagnosis of VT is the presence of atrioventricular dissociation (AVD). Certain leads do not demonstrate AVD to any significant degree (i.e., leads I and V6) while others, simultaneously performed, will demonstrate such a finding as seen here in leads III, V2, and V3. Note the presence of P-waves (arrows) in these leads, signifying AVD and confirming VT.

31. **Wandering atrial pacemaker, rate 92, occasional premature ventricular complexes.** Wandering atrial pacemaker is diagnosed when varying P-waves are present with at least three different morphologies and the resulting rate is <100. The resulting rhythm is irregularly irregular. When the rate is >100/minute, multifocal atrial tachycardia (MAT) is diagnosed. The 3rd and the 15th beats are premature ventricular complexes (PVCs). Much like MAT, wandering pacemaker often occurs in patients with a history of pulmonary disease, and the treatment is based on correcting any underlying conditions (hypoxia, electrolyte abnormalities, etc.). After this patient was treated for an emphysema exacerbation and for mild hypokalemia, the rhythm reverted to SR. See figure opposite.

32. **AV junctional rhythm, rate 48, right bundle branch block (RBBB).** P-waves are not present preceding the QRS complexes, ruling out SR. The escape rhythm is wide-complex, suggesting either an AV junctional rhythm with aberrant conduction versus a ventricular escape rhythm. A rate between 40–60/minute is typical of AV junctional escape rhythms, whereas ventricular escape rhythms are usually 20–40/minute. Small P-waves are noted immediately following the QRS complex ("retrograde P-waves") in some leads, especially in leads I, aVL, and V2, also favoring a junctional rhythm. See figure opposite.

33. **Sinus tachycardia, rate 110, prolonged QT-interval, biatrial enlargement, T-wave abnormality suggestive of diffuse cardiac ischemia versus intracranial hemorrhage.** Biatrial enlargement is diagnosed based on P-waves in the inferior leads which are peaked and have amplitude >2.5 mm (right atrial enlargement) and P-waves in lead V1 with a downward terminal deflection of amplitude >1 mm and with duration >40 msec (left atrial enlargement). Large, broad-based T-wave inversions with a prolonged QT-interval are sometimes found in patients with acute cardiac ischemia, but in the presence of an altered mental status they are highly specific for

This figure corresponds to case #31

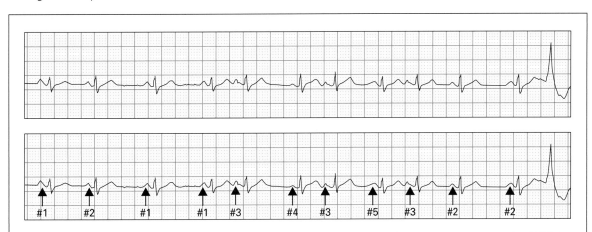

Wandering atrial pacemaker (WAP) is essentially the "slow" version of multifocal atrial tachycardia (MAT). WAP is diagnosed with the demonstration of rates less than 100 beats/minute and at least three different P-wave morphologies within a single ECG lead. The rhythm is irregular.

This figure corresponds to case #32

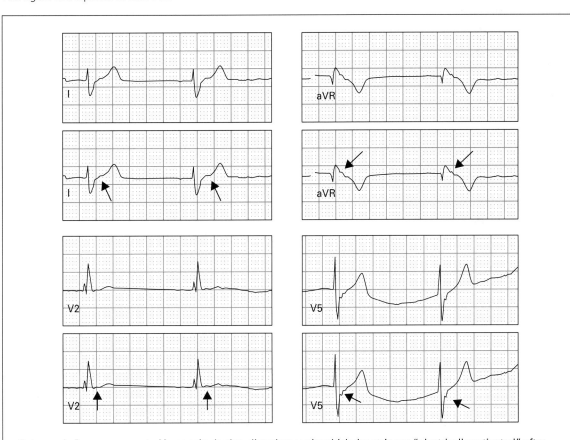

Retrograde P-waves are noted in certain rhythm disturbances in which the atria are "electrically activated" after depolarization of the ventricular myocardium has occurred. In this case, a P-wave can be noted. This P-wave results from a retrograde conduction of the impulse from the AV node to the atrial tissues, producing an atrial depolarization. This retrograde conduction can produce a P-wave which is not always imaged in all leads. As noted in this ECG, only certain leads demonstrate the retrograde P-wave (arrows).

81

elevated intracranial pressure, commonly due to hemorrhage. As a result, this T-wave abnormality is often referred to as a "cerebral T-wave pattern." The exact reason why this intracranial pathology induces the T-wave pattern is debated. Regardless, the ECG distinction between cardiac ischemia versus elevated intracranial pressure is critical, as misdiagnosis can result in inappropriate anticoagulation of a patient with intracranial hemorrhage. This patient had a computed tomogram of the head which demonstrated a hemorrhagic stroke with impending uncal herniation.

34. **Ectopic atrial rhythm, rate 97, acute pericarditis.** Ectopic atrial rhythm is diagnosed because of inverted P-waves in lead III, which excludes the sinus node as the origin of the P-waves. The PR interval is normal, excluding an AV junctional rhythm. Diffuse ST-segment elevation is noted. Causes of diffuse ST-segment elevation include large acute MI, acute pericarditis, benign early repolarization, coronary vasospasm, and LVH. Very subtle PR-segment depression is present several leads (I, II, V4–V6), suggesting acute pericarditis. Additionally, PR-segment elevation is present in lead aVR, and is most suggestive of pericarditis amongst the various entities in the differential diagnosis.

35. **SB with AV junctional escape beats, rate 50.** The underlying rhythm appears to be originating from the sinus node. The first QRS complex on the ECG is preceded by an upright P-wave. The next QRS complex, however, follows a long pause, is narrow, and is without a preceding P-wave. This complex is an AV junctional escape beat caused by the long pause. The pattern is repeated: sinus beat followed by long pause followed by AV junctional escape beat. The overall ventricular rate is approximately 50/minute. This patient had recently started a new calcium channel blocking medication which resulted in the bradycardic rhythm.

36. **SR, rate 60, persistent juvenile T-wave pattern.** Children and teens frequently manifest T-wave inversions in the right precordial leads, V1–V3. This "juvenile T-wave pattern" often persists into young adulthood in women, and may persist even into the 40s. This normal variant is termed "persistent juvenile T-wave pattern." The T-waves in this variant should be asymmetric and shallow in depth and should be limited only to the right precordial leads. If the T-waves are deeply inverted (e.g. >3 mm amplitude), symmetric in shape, extend to V4–V6, or are present in limb leads as well, cardiac ischemia must be assumed.

37. **ST, rate 115, incomplete RBBB, rightward axis, T-wave abnormality consistent with inferior and anteroseptal ischemia, consider acute pulmonary embolism.** Rightward axis can be caused by left posterior fascicular block, right ventricular hypertrophy, lateral MI (if large Q-waves are present), acute (e.g. pulmonary embolism) or chronic (e.g. emphysema) lung disease, ventricular ectopy (i.e. ventricular tachycardia), hyperkalemia, sodium-channel blocking drug toxicity (e.g. cyclic antidepressants), and misplaced leads. In patients with acute cardiopulmonary symptoms, lateral MI, pulmonary embolism, and ventricular tachycardia should be of highest concern. The ECG also demonstrates simultaneous T-wave inversions in the inferior and anteroseptal leads, a combination that has been noted by some authors[1–3] to be highly specific for acute pulmonary hypertension, especially pulmonary embolism, when these ECG findings are new. This patient did, in fact, prove to have a large "saddle" embolism on pulmonary computed tomography.

38. **SB, rate 55, anterolateral ischemia, consider Wellens' syndrome.** In 1982 Wellens and colleagues[4] described two electrocardiographic T-wave abnormalities in leads V2–V4 which had high specificity for critical occlusion of the proximal left anterior descending artery (LAD). The T-waves in this "Wellens' syndrome" demonstrated either deep symmetric inversion or a biphasic morphology (see figure opposite). These patients are often asymptomatic, have no ST-segment changes, and often have normal cardiac biomarkers at initial presentation. Wellens demonstrated that these patients are at high risk for extensive anterior wall MI within 2–3 weeks. This patient's ECG displays Type I Wellens T-waves. Biphasic T-waves are also noted in the inferior leads II and III,

This figure corresponds to case #38

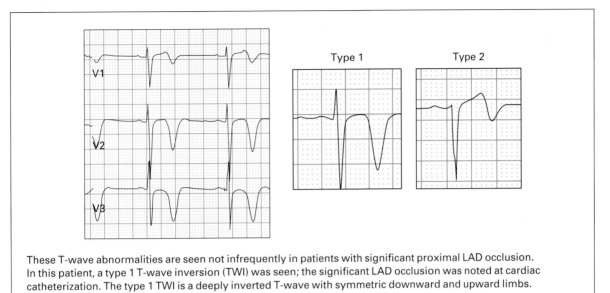

These T-wave abnormalities are seen not infrequently in patients with significant proximal LAD occlusion. In this patient, a type 1 T-wave inversion (TWI) was seen; the significant LAD occlusion was noted at cardiac catheterization. The type 1 TWI is a deeply inverted T-wave with symmetric downward and upward limbs. The type 2 TWI seen in Wellens' syndrome is a biphasic T wave abnormality.

though the significance of this finding is uncertain. The patient was sent for cardiac catheterization and found to have a 90% occlusion of the LAD artery.

39. **ST, rate 105, infero-antero-lateral ischemia, consider left main coronary artery (LMCA) occlusion.** Diffuse ischemia is diagnosed based on the ST-segment depression in multiple leads. Of note, however, is the ST-segment elevation (STE) in lead aVR. In the presence of acute cardiac ischemia, STE in lead aVR is strongly suggestive of occlusion of the LMCA. When the magnitude of the STE in aVR is greater than the STE in lead V1 (as is seen here), or when there is simultaneous STE in leads aVR and aVL, the specificity for LMCA occlusion increases.[5,6] Involvement of the LMCA in ACS is associated with 70% mortality without prompt invasive therapy (percutaneous intervention, bypass surgery). Medical management alone is ineffective. This patient immediately was sent for catheterization and was found to have a 95% occlusion of the LMCA.

40. **ST with first degree AV block, rate 130, RBBB, premature ventricular complexes, acute anterior MI, inferior MI of uncertain age.** The ECG shows evidence of a RBBB, including wide QRS complex (≥120 msec), qR complex in V1, and widening of the S-wave in leads I, V5, and V6. The normal RBBB is also characterized by isoelectric or depressed ST-segments and inverted T-waves in leads V1–V3. In this case, there is marked ST-segment elevation in V1–V5, diagnostic of acute anterior MI. Q-waves have already developed in these leads. The presence of Q-waves in leads II, III, and aVF without ST-segment changes indicates a prior inferior MI of uncertain age. Emergency cardiac catheterization revealed a completely occluded LAD artery.

41. **ST with second degree AV block type II (Mobitz II), ventricular rate 57, occasional PVCs, left ventricular hypertrophy, anterior ischemia.** Sinus tachycardia is diagnosed based on upright P-waves in the limb leads except aVR with an atrial rate of 100/min. The overall ventricular response, however, is significantly less due to the presence of the non-conducted atrial beats of second degree AV block. Although the majority of the rhythm demonstrates second degree AV block with 2:1 conduction (2 P-waves for every 1 QRS complex), the mid-portion of the ECG demonstrates one section of 3:2 conduction. In this small segment of the rhythm, the PR-segment

remains constant, therefore confirming Mobitz II conduction rather than Mobitz I conduction. The second QRS complex on the ECG is a PVC. Leftward axis is present, the differential diagnosis of which includes left anterior fascicular block, LBBB, inferior MI, LVH, ventricular ectopy, paced beats, and Wolff-Parkinson-White syndrome. In this case, LVH accounts for the leftward axis. LVH is diagnosed based on an R-wave in aVL >11 mm. Inverted T-waves are present in the anterior leads, consistent with ischemia.

42. **SR, rate 70, LVH, acute inferior-posterior-lateral MI, probable right ventricular MI.** ST-segment elevation is present in the inferior leads (with early q-wave formation) and lateral precordial leads, consistent with acute inferior and lateral MI. Posterior MI is strongly suggested by the presence of tall R-waves in leads V2–V3. Tall R-waves in the right precordial leads in the setting of an acute MI are analogous to q-waves, or infarction, in the posterior region of the heart. Right ventricular extension of an inferior MI is strongly suggested when the magnitude of ST-segment elevation in lead III is significantly greater than the ST-segment elevation in lead II, as is the case here. Approximately one-third of inferior MIs will extend to the posterior region of the heart, and one-third will extend to the right ventricle (RV). Posterior extension of the MI can be confirmed by placement of additional leads in the left mid-back area just inferior to the inferior pole of the scapula. When the ECG is repeated with these posterior leads, acute posterior MI demonstrates typical acute MI findings of q-wave formation and STE in those leads. RV extension of the MI can be confirmed by placing precordial leads across the right side of the chest (mirror image of their normal left-sided placement) and then repeating the ECG. RV MI will then demonstrate ST-segment elevation in those right precordial leads. LVH is diagnosed based on the presence of an R-wave in lead aVL >11 mm in height. See figure below.

This figure corresponds to case #42

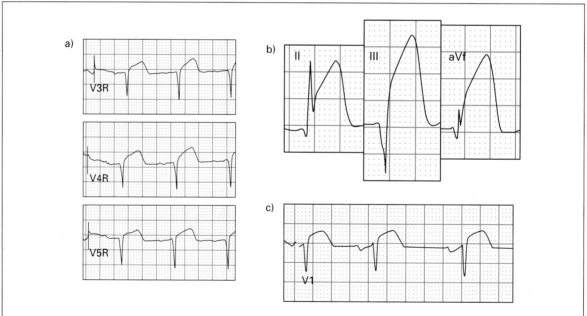

Right ventricular (RV) myocardial infarction most often occurs in the setting of inferior wall acute MI—of note, approximately 30% of patients with inferior wall MI will also suffer an RV infarction. In this setting, clinical and electrocardiographic findings will suggest the diagnosis. Clinically, systemic hypotension spontaneously or after a vasodilating agent (nitroglycerin or morphine) with clear lung fields suggests RV infarction. Electrocardiographically, numerous findings are supportive of RV infarction in the setting of an inferior wall MI. a) Right-sided ECG leads will demonstrate STE. b) Disproportionate ST-segment elevation in lead III relative to leads II and aVF. c) ST-segment elevation in lead V1.

43. **SR with first degree AV block, rate 60, occasional PVCs, non-specific intraventricular conduction delay, digitalis effect.** The PR interval is >200 msec, consistent with a first degree AV block. Digitalis effect is diagnosed based on the sagging ST-segment depression with upward concavity noted in many of the leads, especially leads V4–V6. This ST-segment depression creates a characteristic appearance of the terminal portion of the QRS complex resembling the end of a hockey-stick (many refer to this as a "Salvador Dali moustache" appearance). Although this morphology only suggests the *presence* of digitalis, mild *toxicity* is suspected based on the slow heart rate, first degree AV block, and PVCs. PVCs are the most common ECG manifestation of digitalis toxicity, although they are non-specific. This patient was suffering from mild chronic digoxin toxicity (level 3.3 ng/mL; normal level is 0.5–2.2 ng/mL). A non-specific intraventricular conduction delay (IVCD) is diagnosed based on a slightly wide QRS complex (duration is 114 msec) which does not meet the criteria for any of the other typical causes of QRS prolongation (hypothermia, hyperkalemia, WPW, BBB, ventricular ectopy). See figure below.

This figure corresponds to case #43. Digoxin effect

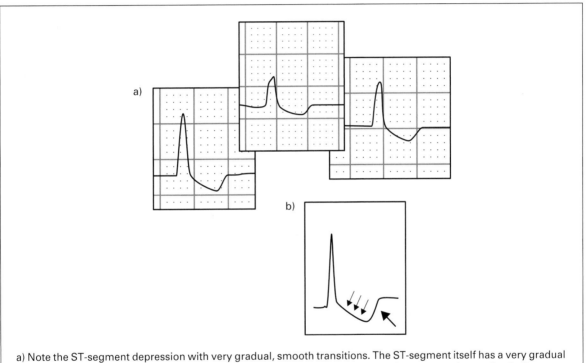

a) Note the ST-segment depression with very gradual, smooth transitions. The ST-segment itself has a very gradual downsloping limb coupled with a more abrupt upsloping portion. This form of ST-segment depression indicates only the presence of a digitalis compound in the systemic circulation. It is not necessarily indicative of *toxicity*.
b) The small arrows indicate the gradual downward limb and the large arrow, the more abrupt return to the baseline.

44. **SR, rate 75, acute inferior-posterior-lateral MI.** Baseline artifact on the ECG causes some difficulty in rhythm interpretation, but the lead II rhythm strip does appear to show a sinus rhythm. ST-segment elevation is noted in the inferior and lateral leads consistent with acute MI. Posterior extension is suspected based on (1) ST-segment depression (although minor) in leads V1–V3, (2) large R-waves in leads V2–V3, and (3) relatively tall upright T-waves in leads V2–V3. These findings in the presence of a concurrent inferior MI should always prompt consideration of posterior extension of the MI. Placement of posterior leads can help clarify whether posterior MI is present. In this case, three leads labeled V7, V8, and V9 were placed on the patient's left mid-back area inferior to the lower pole of the scapula, and the ECG was repeated. In these posterior leads, STE is noted, thus confirming posterior MI. See figure on p. 86.

This figure corresponds to case #44. Posterior wall myocardial infarction

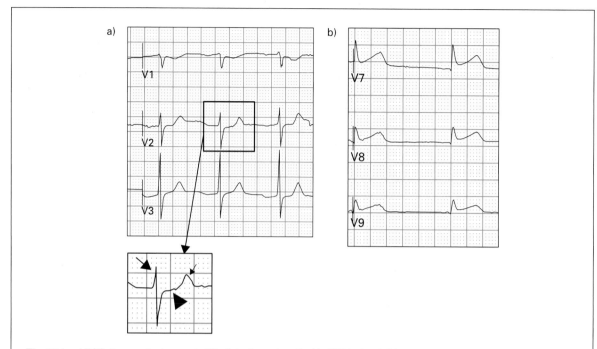

The 12-lead ECG demonstrates acute MI of the lateral wall with STE in leads V5 and V6; subtle changes of the ST-segment waveform in lead II suggest the possibility of an inferior event as well. a) In leads V1 to V3, a posterior wall MI is suggested. Note that these anterior leads also image the posterior wall indirectly. Suggested findings of posterior wall MI in these leads includes prominent R-wave (large arrow), ST-segment depression (arrowhead), and upright T-waves (small arrow). b) Posterior ECG leads demonstrating STE, indicative of an acute posterior wall MI.

45. **SR with second degree AV block type I (Wenckebach, Mobitz I), rate 55, non-specific IVCD.** The rhythm was originally misdiagnosed as atrial fibrillation because of the baseline artifact and the slight irregularity of the rhythm. However, closer inspection does reveal regular atrial activity. Distinct P-waves are most easily found in lead V1, excluding the diagnosis of atrial fibrillation. Close inspection of the lead II rhythm strip reveals regular atrial activity and gradual prolongation of the PR interval until a non-conducted P-wave appears. The cycle then repeats. Some of the P-wave are hidden within T-waves. Non-specific IVCD is diagnosed based on the presence of slight QRS complex prolongation without meeting formal criteria of any of the usual causes of a prolonged QRS interval (hypothermia, hyperkalemia, WPW, bundle branch block, ventricular ectopy, paced beats, LVH, and sodium channel blocking medications).

46. **SR with high-grade AV block, rate 50, LVH.** The atrial rate is 88 but the ventricular rate is only 50, indicating the presence of an AV block. There does not appear to be a regular association between the P-waves and QRS complexes. While some of the QRS complexes follow a relatively normal PR interval and appear to be conducted beats, other QRS complexes appear more isolated (e.g. the first QRS complex) and may be escape beats. Additionally, many of the P-waves are non-conducted. The rhythm does not meet criteria for diagnosis as second degree or third degree (complete) heart block, and as a result is simply referred to as "high-grade AV block." This patient did go on to develop complete heart block but recovered in time. He was eventually diagnosed with Lyme carditis.

47. **ST, rate 110, right ventricular hypertrophy (RVH), T-wave abnormality consistent with inferior and anteroseptal ischemia, consider acute pulmonary embolism.** There are many ECG manifestations associated with acute pulmonary embolism (PE), including sinus tachycardia rightward axis, tall R-waves in the right precordial leads (often attributed to right heart strain), T-wave inversions, and of course the "classic" $S_IQ_{III}T_{III}$ (large S in lead I, Q-wave in lead III, and T-wave inversion in lead III). The majority of these findings have been found to be neither sensitive nor specific. However, as noted previously, the combination of T-wave inversions in the inferior and the anteroseptal leads has been described as highly specific for acute pulmonary hypertension, often the result of acute PE. Further supporting the diagnosis of acute PE in this patient is the presence of a rightward axis (differential diagnosis includes left posterior fascicular block, right ventricular hypertrophy, lateral MI, acute pulmonary embolism, emphysema, ventricular ectopy, hyperkalemia, sodium-channel blocking drug toxicity, and misplaced leads). Right ventricular hypertrophy is diagnosed by the presence of rightward axis, tall R-wave in lead V1 ≥7 mm, and qR pattern in lead V1. This patient had developed RVH and pulmonary hypertension because of multiple prior PEs. During this current episode, she developed a saddle embolus and died soon after her arrival in the emergency department.

This figure corresponds to case #47. Electrocardiographic findings suggestive of pulmonary embolism include sinus tachycardia, right ventricular hypertrophy (RVH) and the classic $S_IQ_{III}T_{III}$ pattern

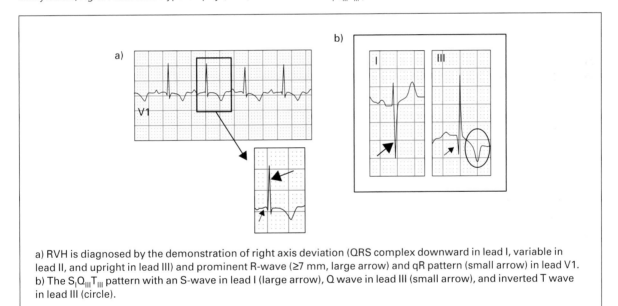

a) RVH is diagnosed by the demonstration of right axis deviation (QRS complex downward in lead I, variable in lead II, and upright in lead III) and prominent R-wave (≥7 mm, large arrow) and qR pattern (small arrow) in lead V1.
b) The $S_IQ_{III}T_{III}$ pattern with an S-wave in lead I (large arrow), Q wave in lead III (small arrow), and inverted T wave in lead III (circle).

48. **SR, rate 70, J-waves suggestive of hypothermia.** Baseline artifact is noted because the patient was shivering—the patient's body temperature was 30 degrees Celsius (86 degrees Fahrenheit). Osborne waves (also known as "J waves") are usually most notable in the precordial leads, although in this case they are present in limb leads as well. They actually appear inverted in leads V1–V2 in this case. Osborne waves are characteristic of hypothermia, although they are not pathognomonic. Other common ECG findings in patients with hypothermia, although not present in this case, include prolongation of the intervals, bradycardias and AV blocks, and ventricular arrhythmias. As this patient was warmed, the Osborne waves became less prominent and finally resolved by the time he was 34 degrees Celsius (93.2 degrees Fahrenheit).

49.	**SR with second degree AV block type 2 (Mobitz II), rate 47, probable reversal of leads V2 and V3.** Second degree AV block is characterized by intermittent non-conducted P-waves. Mobitz II conduction is diagnosed when the PR-intervals in the conducted beats remain constant. The R-wave progression in the anteroseptal leads is abnormal, and is likely the result of reversed positions of leads V2 and V3 on the chest wall.

50.	**SR, rate 60, T-wave abnormality suggestive of hypokalemia.** ECG findings typically associated with hypokalemia include U-waves, ventricular ectopy, ST-segment depression, and T-wave flattening. In the authors' experience, moderate-to-severe hypokalemia often induces an unusual biphasic T-wave appearance in the mid-precordial leads as noted in this example. The ST-segment sags downwards, often producing frank ST-segment depression, then rises into an upright T-wave with a slightly prolonged overall QT interval. It may be that this upright T-wave is actually a U-wave following an inverted T-wave. Regardless, this biphasic complex is character-istic of hypokalemia and resolves with appropriate treatment. This patient's serum potassium level was 2.9 mEq/L (normal 3.5–5.3 mEq/L). The biphasic T-wave of hypokalemia should not be confused with the biphasic T-wave found in Wellens' syndrome, in which the initial portion of the T-wave rises and the terminal portion inverts. Essentially, they are mirror images of each other.

51.	**ST with first degree AV block, rate 100, LAFB, septal infarct of uncertain age, inferior and anterior ischemia, consider LMCA occlusion.** LAFB is diagnosed based on the leftward axis, the qR complexes in I and aVL, and the rS complexes in III. Q-waves present in leads V1–V2 indicated a septal infarct of uncertain age. ST-segment depression is present in the inferior and anterior leads and T-wave inversions are present in the lateral leads, overall suggesting diffuse ischemia. Of greatest concern, however, is evidence suggesting occlusion of the left LMCA: ST-segment elevation simultaneously in leads aVR and aVL; and also STE in lead aVR greater in magnitude than the STE in lead V1. The presence of either of these two findings alone is strongly suggestive of LMCA occlusion. Occlusion of the LMCA in the setting of an acute coronary syndrome portends a 70% mortality unless prompt invasive therapy is instituted. Unfortunately, this patient died before he could be taken for coro-nary intervention.

52.	**SR, rate 95, high left ventricular voltage (HLVV), acute pericarditis.** The term "high left ventricular voltage" is used when large amplitude QRS complexes are present in young patients. Generally, left ventricular hypertro-phy (LVH) should not be diagnosed in patients <40–45 years of age purely based on large amplitude QRS complexes. LVH represents a pathologic condition, whereas "high left ventricular voltage" simply represents a normal variant and is common in healthy young patients, especially athletes. Diffuse STE is present. Amongst the various conditions that are well-known to produce diffuse ST-segment elevation (large AMI, acute pericar-ditis, benign early repolarization, ventricular aneurysm, coronary vasospasm), pericarditis is the only one in which PR-segment depression is found. In this ECG, PR-segment depression is noted in the inferior and anterior leads. Two other findings are suggestive of pericarditis as well: there is PR-segment elevation in lead aVR, and the magnitude of the STE in lead II is greater than that found in lead III. Neither of these two findings are 100% specific for pericarditis, however, and care should be taken to avoid over-relying on these findings alone in ruling out AMI. See figure opposite.

53.	**SR, rate 80, HLVV, acute septal MI, consider LMCA occlusion.** The concave upward morphology of the ST segments in leads V1–V2, especially in a 28 year old man, is suggestive of a benign form of STE. However, given the presence of ST-segment depression in multiple leads, the necessary assumption is that the STE in leads V1–V2 must represent AMI. Furthermore, concurrent STE in leads aVR and aVL is highly specific for LMCA occlusion. This young man, who had no prior-known atherosclerotic risk factors, was transferred immediately for percutaneous coronary intervention (PCI) and was found to have diffuse atherosclerotic disease including critical occlusions of

This figure corresponds to case #52

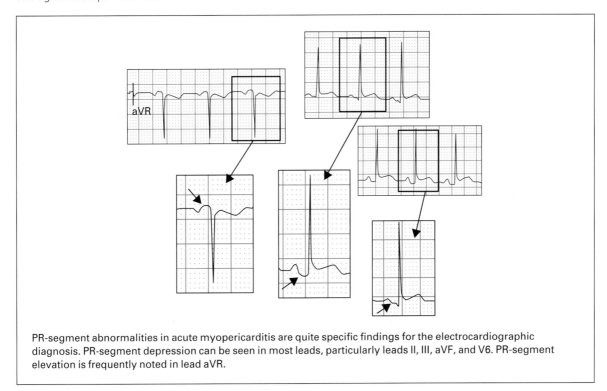

PR-segment abnormalities in acute myopericarditis are quite specific findings for the electrocardiographic diagnosis. PR-segment depression can be seen in most leads, particularly leads II, III, aVF, and V6. PR-segment elevation is frequently noted in lead aVR.

the LAD artery and LMCA. He developed cardiogenic shock and required placement of a balloon pump for hemodynamic support, but he survived.

54. **Atrial fibrillation with rapid ventricular response, rate 170, bifascicular block (RBBB and LAFB), LVH, lateral ischemia.** The three main diagnostic considerations with irregularly irregular tachycardias are atrial fibrillation, multifocal atrial tachycardia, and atrial flutter with variable AV conduction. The latter two diagnoses are characterized by discernable P-waves, which are absent in this case. Widening of the QRS complex is caused by a RBBB, diagnosed based on the presence of an rsR' pattern in the right precordial leads and a wide S-wave in the lateral leads I, V5–V6. LAFB is also diagnosed based on the leftward axis, the qR complexes in I and aVL, and rS complexes in III. LVH is diagnosed based on the R-wave amplitude in aVL >11 mm. Whereas slight ST-segment depression in the right precordial leads may be a normal finding in the presence of RBBB, the ST-segment depression noted in the lateral leads V4–V6 is not normal, and suggests lateral ischemia. See figure on p. 90.

55. **Ventricular tachycardia (VT), rate 145.** The three main diagnostic considerations with regular wide QRS complex tachycardias are VT, SVT with aberrant conduction, and ST with aberrant conduction. In the absence of a regular P-QRS relationship indicating ST, VT should always be assumed. SVT with aberrant conduction should only be a diagnosis of absolute exclusion. In this case, the presence of a rightward axis and history of recent cardiac arrest is highly specific for VT. Retrograde P-waves are sometimes noted with VT, and are present in this case—lead II, especially, demonstrates P-waves embedded in the terminal portion of the QRS complexes.

This figure corresponds to case #54. Atrial fibrillation with rapid ventricular response and abnormally widened QRS complex

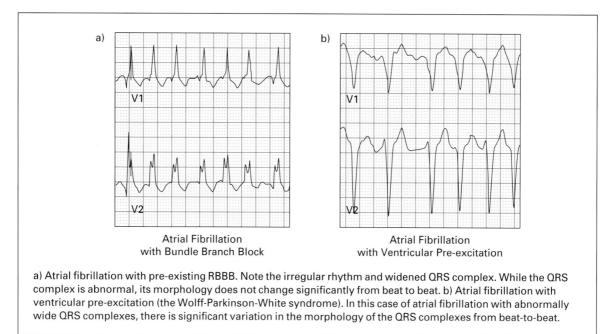

a)

b)

Atrial Fibrillation
with Bundle Branch Block

Atrial Fibrillation
with Ventricular Pre-excitation

a) Atrial fibrillation with pre-existing RBBB. Note the irregular rhythm and widened QRS complex. While the QRS complex is abnormal, its morphology does not change significantly from beat to beat. b) Atrial fibrillation with ventricular pre-excitation (the Wolff-Parkinson-White syndrome). In this case of atrial fibrillation with abnormally wide QRS complexes, there is significant variation in the morphology of the QRS complexes from beat-to-beat.

56. **SR with second degree AV block type 1 (Mobitz I, Wenckebach), rate 60, HLVV, benign early repolarization (BER).** Mobitz I is characterized by regular P-waves (here, the atrial rate is approximately 80/min and regular) with progressive prolongation of the PR-interval until a P-wave fails to conduct to the ventricle, producing a pause in the ventricular response. STE is noted in leads V2–V4. The presence of a slight upstroke at the end of the QRS complex in leads V3–V4 and lead II, producing what is sometimes referred to as a "fishhook appearance" at the end of the QRS complex, is characteristic of BER. Acute MI and BER can sometimes be confused. Helpful clues that distinguish acute MI and exclude BER include the presence of reciprocal ST-segment depression in some leads, any convex upward ST-segment elevation, or evolving changes noted on serial ECGs. Additionally, the STE of BER is rare in the elderly, especially elderly women, and usually localized to the anterior and lateral precordial leads.

57. **ST with first degree AV block, rate 105, LAFB, non-specific intraventricular conduction delay (IVCD) and prominent T-waves suggestive of hyperkalemia.** The well-known ECG manifestations of hyperkalemia include prominent, peaked T-waves and widening of the QRS complex (non-specific IVCD). Hyperkalemia is also well-known to produce new fascicular blocks, bundle branch blocks, AV blocks and flattening of the P-wave. At advanced stages of hyperkalemia, the P-waves become flat and often cannot be found within the tracing. In this example, hyperkalemia has induced a first degree AV block and flattened, barely noticeable P-waves. This patient's dehydration had caused new renal failure and hyperkalemia. His serum potassium level was 8.0 mEq/L (normal 3.5–5.3 mEq/L). See figure opposite.

This figure corresponds to case #57

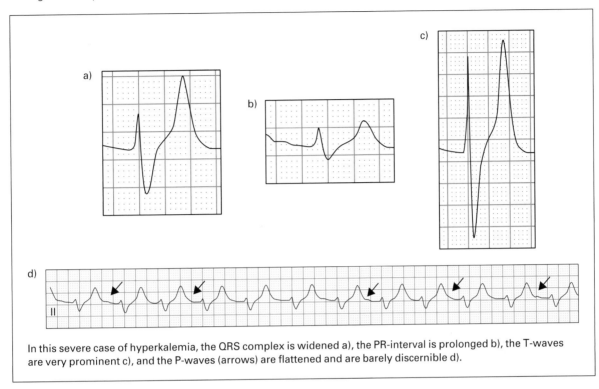

In this severe case of hyperkalemia, the QRS complex is widened a), the PR-interval is prolonged b), the T-waves are very prominent c), and the P-waves (arrows) are flattened and are barely discernible d).

58. **Polymorphic VT, probable torsade de pointes, rate 250.** The rhythm is a wide complex tachycardia with varying QRS morphologies. The two main diagnostic considerations in this setting are polymorphic ventricular tachycardia and atrial fibrillation with Wolff-Parkinson-White syndrome. The latter, however, tends to be much more irregular, whereas in this case the rhythm is fairly regular. Torsade de pointes is a specific type of polymorphic VT that is associated with prolonged QT during sinus rhythm; and it has a characteristic rhythmic appearance of the QRS complexes, which gradually vary from larger to smaller and back again in amplitude, and they also gradually change in axis. Formal diagnosis of torsade de pointes would require an ECG in sinus rhythm demonstrating a prolonged QT interval. This patient did, in fact, demonstrate a prolonged QT interval on his baseline ECG. He had recently increased his dosage of methadone, a medication known to prolong the QT interval.

59. **SB, rate 45, acute lateral MI.** The ECG leads which correspond to the lateral wall of the left ventricle are I, aVL, V5, and V6. Leads I and aVL, more specifically, correspond to the high lateral portion of the left ventricle. Although these two leads are not adjacent to each other on the ECG, they *are* considered "contiguous" leads for purposes of acute reperfusion therapy. This patient has STE in leads I and aVL and, therefore, is a candidate for acute reperfusion therapy (immediate PCI or fibrinolytics) for acute STE MI. ST-segment depression representing reciprocal change is noted in leads III and aVF. Inferior leads II and aVF, similar to lateral leads I and aVL, are also considered contiguous leads despite the fact that they are not adjacent to each other on the ECG.

60. **Multifocal atrial tachycardia (MAT), rate 115, LVH, diffuse ischemia.** When the rhythm is an irregularly irregular tachycardia, the main diagnostic considerations are atrial fibrillation, atrial flutter with variable AV conduction, and MAT. The presence of distinct P-waves excludes the diagnosis of atrial fibrillation. On the contrary, P-waves are present with at least three different morphologies and they occur at irregular intervals, confirming the diagnosis of MAT and excluding the diagnosis of atrial flutter. MAT is often associated with pulmonary disease—this patient was suffering from an acute exacerbation of emphysema. Slight ST-segment depression is noted in multiple leads and resolved with treatment of the patient's hypoxia.

61. **SR with PACs in a pattern of atrial bigeminy, rate 75, non-specific intraventricular conduction delay.** The QRS complexes appear in groups of two, separated by brief pauses, creating a regularly irregular rhythm. The presence of grouped beats, or regular irregularity, is usually the result of either PACs or second degree AV block (Mobitz I or II). In this case, the second QRS in each group is preceded by a P-wave that differs in morphology from its predecessor. This second P-QRS complex is also followed by a short pause. This is characteristic of a PAC. In fact, the most common overall cause of a pause in the cardiac rhythm is a preceding PAC. When every second QRS complex is the result of a PAC, atrial bigeminy is diagnosed. The QRS complexes are markedly wide. The differential diagnosis of wide QRS complexes includes hypothermia, hyperkalemia, WPW, aberrant ventricular conduction (e.g. bundle branch block), ventricular ectopy, paced beats, and certain medications. In the absence of diagnostic criteria for any of the above, the term "non-specific intraventricular conduction delay" is used. Although the QRS complexes resemble a LBBB, the presence of q-waves, even small ones, in the lateral leads excludes the diagnosis of LBBB. See figure below.

This figure corresponds to case #61. Premature atrial contractions in a bigeminy pattern

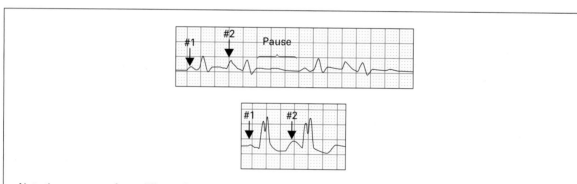

Note the presence of two different P-wave morphologies (#1 and #2) as well as the compensatory pause. P-wave #1 likely results from a sinus node-originated beat while P-wave #2 results from an ectopic atrial focus.

62. **SR, rate 64, LAFB, LVH, prolonged QT-interval, T-wave abnormality suggestive of diffuse cardiac ischemia versus intracranial hemorrhage.** The most prominent abnormality is the presence of giant T-wave inversions in the precordial leads. T-wave inversions of this magnitude in patients with a depressed level of consciousness are highly suggestive of a large intracranial hemorrhage, and in fact are often referred to as "cerebral T-wave pattern." These T-wave abnormalities may be present in the setting of non-hemorrhagic cerebral disorders as well (e.g. cerebral edema, ischemic stroke), but less commonly. They may be present in the limb leads, although they tend to be most prominent in the precordial leads where their magnitude may be up to 20 mm or more. A prolonged QT-interval is typically associated with these "cerebral T-waves." Rarely T-wave inversions of this magnitude may occur in the setting of cardiac ischemia, but those patients are likely to have a normal mental status. The exact reason why cerebral disorders can cause these unusual T-waves is uncertain. This patient did in fact have a large intracranial hemorrhage and died within two days. See figure opposite.

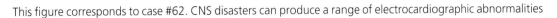

This figure corresponds to case #62. CNS disasters can produce a range of electrocardiographic abnormalities

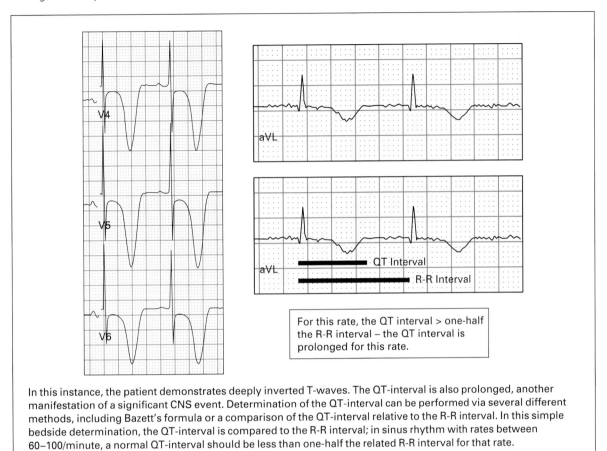

aVL

aVL QT Interval

R-R Interval

For this rate, the QT interval > one-half the R-R interval – the QT interval is prolonged for this rate.

In this instance, the patient demonstrates deeply inverted T-waves. The QT-interval is also prolonged, another manifestation of a significant CNS event. Determination of the QT-interval can be performed via several different methods, including Bazett's formula or a comparison of the QT-interval relative to the R-R interval. In this simple bedside determination, the QT-interval is compared to the R-R interval; in sinus rhythm with rates between 60–100/minute, a normal QT-interval should be less than one-half the related R-R interval for that rate.

63. **SR with second degree AV block type 1 (Wenckebach, Mobitz I), rate 50, LBBB.** The atrial rate is approximately 60, although the approximate ventricular rate is 50. Non-conducted P-waves are present and a constant P-P interval persists, indicating the presence of an AV block. For those P-waves that are conducted, the PR interval appears to gradually increase preceding the non-conducted P-waves. The increasing PR interval defines Mobitz I AV conduction. The novice interpreter may miss the non-conducted P-waves because both of the non-conducted P-waves on the rhythm strip are "buried" within the T-waves. A LBBB is also present with expected ST-segment discordance—ST-segments are *normally* deviated opposite to the terminal deflection of the QRS complex when a LBBB is present (i.e. when the terminal portion of the QRS complex points primarily upwards, ST-segment depression is expected; when the terminal portion of the QRS complex points downwards, STE is expected). See figure on p. 94.

64. **Ventricular tachycardia (VT), rate 190.** The differential diagnosis of a wide QRS complex tachycardia includes VT, SVT with aberrant conduction (e.g. bundle branch block), and ST with aberrant conduction. In the absence of an obvious and repeating P-QRS pattern, ST can be excluded. This patient's ECG does demonstrate several features which exclude the diagnosis of SVT and confirm VT: a taller left "rabbit ear" morphology of the QRS complex in lead V1, S > R in lead V6, AV dissociation, and the presence of fusion complexes. Even in the absence of these diagnostic features, however, VT should always be preferentially chosen and treated rather than SVT—treatment of an SVT as if it were VT is generally safe; however, if VT is mistakenly diagnosed and treated as SVT, the results can be deadly. See figure on p. 94.

This figure corresponds to case #63

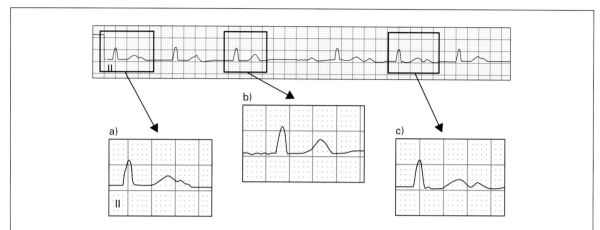

The P-waves are partially obscured by the T-wave in a) and c); the P-wave is entirely obscured by the T-wave in this beat b).

This figure corresponds to case #64. Features suggestive of VT in this wide QRS complex tachycardia

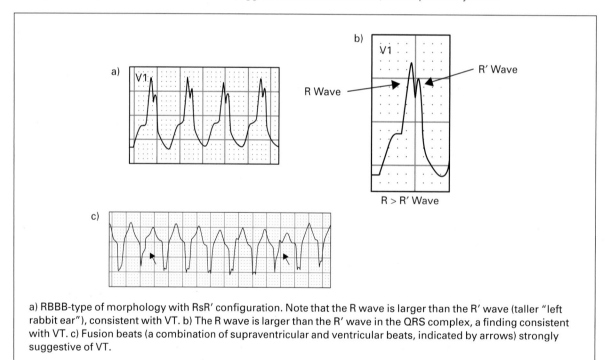

a) RBBB-type of morphology with RsR' configuration. Note that the R wave is larger than the R' wave (taller "left rabbit ear"), consistent with VT. b) The R wave is larger than the R' wave in the QRS complex, a finding consistent with VT. c) Fusion beats (a combination of supraventricular and ventricular beats, indicated by arrows) strongly suggestive of VT.

65. **SR with first degree AV block, rate 70, possible inferior-posterior-lateral MI of undetermined age, non-specific IVCD, LVH, T-wave abnormality suggestive of hyperkalemia**. In the absence of further clinical information, the ECG is confusing. A prominent R-wave is present in lead V1 and the QRS progression across the precordium is unusual. The differential diagnosis for this finding includes WPW, posterior MI, RBBB (or incomplete RBBB), ventricular ectopy, right ventricular hypertrophy, acute right ventricular dilatation (right ventricular "strain," e.g. massive pulmonary embolism), hypertrophic cardiomyopathy, progressive muscular dystrophy, dextrocardia, and misplaced precordial electrodes. Small q-waves are present in the inferior and lateral leads suggestive of a prior MI and lend credence to the possibility that the prominent R-wave in lead V1 represents posterior extension of an MI. However, the q-waves are smaller and narrower than normal infarction-induced q-waves—infarction q-waves are expected to be at least 40 msec in duration and at least 25% of the amplitude of the entire QRS complex. Alas, further history and examination solved the puzzle: the patient had a history of **dextrocardia**. When the ECG leads were repositioned to account for this, the small q-waves "disappeared" and the QRS progression "normalized." The prolonged PR interval and the "peaked" T-waves in the precordial leads suggest hyperkalemia. This patient's serum potassium level was 7.9 mEq/L (normal 3.5–5.3 mEq/L). It is important to remember that peaked T-waves of hyperkalemia can be upright *or inverted*, depending on the patient's baseline T-wave morphology.

66. **Probable SB, rate 45, Osborne waves consistent with hypothermia, non-specific T-wave flattening.** Significant artifact (due to shivering) is present, which somewhat obscures rhythm interpretation. However, there appear to be upright P-waves preceding the QRS complexes, best noted in the rhythm strip, consistent with SB. Sizeable upward deflections occur just after the QRS complexes. These are referred to as Osborne waves, or J-waves, and are most notably found in the setting of hypothermia. They tend to be most prominent in the precordial leads, and they gradually reduce in size and eventually disappear with rewarming. This patient's core body temperature was 29 degrees Celsius (84.2 degrees Fahrenheit). Typical ECG abnormalities associated with hypothermia include Osborne waves, sinus bradycardia or atrial fibrillation with slow ventricular response, and prolongation of all of the intervals (PR, QRS, QT). See figure on p. 96.

67. **SR, rate 84, acute pericarditis.** Diffuse STE is present on this ECG. Although there are many conditions that can induce STE on the ECG, the major diagnostic considerations in patients with *diffuse* STE are large AMI, acute pericarditis, BER, and LVH. LVH can be excluded by lack of voltage criteria. Of the remaining three considerations, acute pericarditis is the only one that causes PR-segment depression/downsloping, which is found in leads I and in the anterior and lateral precordial leads.

68. **Accelerated junctional tachycardia, rate 115, bifascicular block (RBBB and LAFB), prolonged QT-interval.** Subtle P-waves are noted on the rhythm strip. However, the PR interval is too short (<120 msec) for normal sinus rhythm unless an accessory pathway were present. There is no evidence of an accessory pathway. The most likely alternative cause of such a short PR interval is a junctional rhythm. A normal AV junctional rate is 40–60 beats/min; thus this is referred to as an *accelerated* junctional tachycardia. A RBBB (QRS duration >120 msec, rsR′ pattern in lead V1, wide S-waves in the lateral leads) and LAFB (leftward axis, rS pattern in lead III and qR in I and aVL) are present as well. This patient was initially misdiagnosed as having sinus tachycardia. He was treated for several hours with intravenous fluids with the assumption that the tachycardia was due to hypovolemia. When his rate showed no evidence of improvement, the proper diagnosis was finally made. He then received a small dose of a beta-blocker medication and immediately converted to sinus rhythm with a rate of 75.

69. **ST with first degree AV block, rate 130, acute inferior-lateral MI with possible posterior MI, anteroseptal MI of undetermined age, prolonged QT-interval.** STE is present in the inferior and lateral leads consistent with AMI. Pronounced ST-segment depression is present in leads V1–V3. In the presence of an inferior AMI,

This figure corresponds to case #66. The electrocardiographic triad of hypothermia: Osborne wave, bradycardia, and artifact

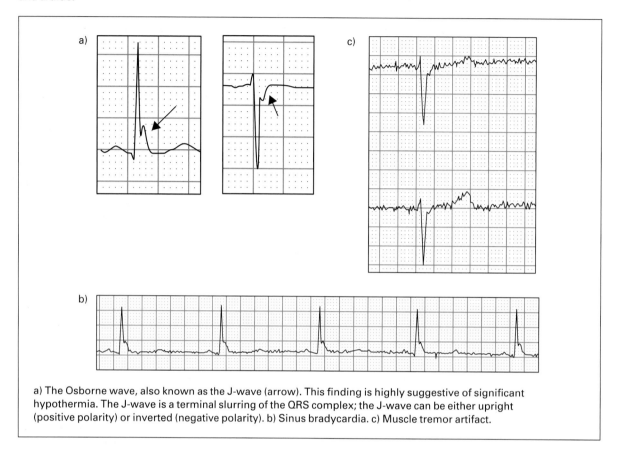

a) The Osborne wave, also known as the J-wave (arrow). This finding is highly suggestive of significant hypothermia. The J-wave is a terminal slurring of the QRS complex; the J-wave can be either upright (positive polarity) or inverted (negative polarity). b) Sinus bradycardia. c) Muscle tremor artifact.

ST-segment depression in the anteroseptal leads can represent either reciprocal change or it can indicate acute posterior MI. Reciprocal ST-segment depression is usually shallow and downsloping, whereas ST-segment depression due to acute posterior MI is usually horizontal and >2 mm depressed. Therefore, the ST-segment depression in this case appears more likely to be due to acute posterior MI. Another expected finding in posterior MI is large R-waves in leads V1–V3. In this case, however, large Q-waves presumably from a prior anteroseptal MI prevent the development of large R-waves. Confirmation of acute posterior MI could be accomplished by repeating the ECG with posterior leads and finding STE. A slightly prolonged QT-interval is also present, and may be caused by acute cardiac ischemia. Other possible causes of QT-interval prolongation include hypokalemia, hypomagnesemia, hypocalcemia, elevated intracranial pressure, drugs with sodium channel blocking effects, hypothermia, and congenital prolonged QT syndrome.

70. **SR, rate 84, occasional premature atrial contractions (PACs), T-wave abnormality and prolonged QT-interval consistent with diffuse ischemia versus hypokalemia.** Hypokalemia can cause an assortment of ECG abnormalities, including atrial or ventricular ectopy, U-waves, and T-wave flattening. Severe hypokalemia can also cause ST-segment sagging that mimics cardiac ischemia, as well as a characteristic biphasic T-wave abnormality in which the initial portion of the T-wave inverts and is followed by an upward deflection. The abnormality is most prominent in the precordial leads. The overall complex produces a prolonged QT-interval. In reality, this complex is actually caused by the fusion of an inverted T-wave with an upright U-wave. This patient was

suffering from alcoholic ketoacidosis, and she had profound hypokalemia (serum level 1.7 mEq/L; normal 3.5–5.3 mEq/L) and hypomagnesemia (serum level 1.0 mg/dL; normal 1.8–2.4 mg/dL). Hypomagnesemia is another cause of prolongation of the QT-interval. The ninth and twelfth QRS complexes are PACs. The PACs as well as the ST-segment depression and the T-wave abnormality resolved after correction of the electrolyte abnormalities.

71. **SR with second degree AV block type 1 (Wenckebach, Mobitz I), rate 50, RBBB.** The atrial rate is approximately 88, and there are frequent non-conducted P-waves that result in an overall ventricular rate of 50. A second degree AV block is present mostly with a 2:1 conduction ratio (two P-waves for every one QRS). When 2:1 conduction occurs, it is impossible to determine with certainty whether the rhythm is Mobitz I or Mobitz II. In this case, however, 3:2 conduction occurs in two portions of the rhythm strip: in the 5th–6th ventricular beats and in the 8th–9th ventricular beats. In these two areas, the PR-interval increases. This confirms the diagnosis of Mobitz I.

72. **SR with wandering pacemaker, rate 85, occasional PVC, non-specific T-wave flattening.** "Wandering pacemaker" is diagnosed when there are at least three separate P-wave morphologies indicating multiple atrial foci that are sending impulses to the ventricle. Essentially this is a slower form of MAT, and much like MAT, it tends to occur in patients with pulmonary disease. Both the atrial and the ventricular ectopy in this case resolved as the patient's asthma exacerbation improved.

73. **Atrial fibrillation, ventricular rate 155, acute anterior-lateral MI, inferior MI of undetermined age.** When a tachydysrhythmia is irregularly irregular, the differential diagnosis is primarily limited to atrial fibrillation, atrial flutter with variable AV conduction, and MAT. The latter two entities should demonstrate distinct atrial activity, which this ECG does not; therefore, the diagnosis of atrial fibrillation is made. STE is present in the mid and lateral precordial leads as well as in leads I and aVL, consistent with AMI. Q-waves have already appeared in a majority of these leads indicating that the duration of ischemia is likely to have been ongoing for at least a few hours (generally considered the minimal time required for the development of infarction-related Q-waves). Q-waves are also present in the inferior leads. Leads III and aVF lack STE, indicating that the Q-waves in those leads are more likely to be from a prior MI rather than acute MI. Lead II, although primarily reflecting the inferior portion of the heart, also provides some information about the lateral areas as well; therefore, the slight STE noted in lead II is probably the result of the acute lateral MI. A leftward axis is present and can be attributed to the prior inferior MI. Other causes of a leftward axis include LBBB, LAFB, LVH, ventricular ectopy, paced beats, and WPW syndrome.

74. **Atrial fibrillation, ventricular rate 100, diffuse ischemia, possible acute posterior MI.** The irregularly irregular rhythm in the absence of distinct atrial activity is likely atrial fibrillation. ST-segment depression is noted in the inferior, anterior, and lateral leads consistent with diffuse ischemia. Tall R-waves in the right precordial leads with large upright T-waves are characteristic of posterior MI, although the expected horizontal ST-segment depression in leads V1–V2 is absent. Posterior leads could help clarify whether the patient was having an acute posterior wall MI but they were not done. This patient had overdosed on heroin and suffered a respiratory arrest followed by cardiac arrest. During the prehospital resuscitation, he received a total of 3 mg of atropine, 3 mg of epinephrine, sodium bicarbonate, dextrose, and naloxone. The ischemic changes noted in this ECG could be related to intrinsic cardiac ischemia, but they could also be related to ischemia resulting from the resuscitation efforts, especially the epinephrine. Epinephrine is well-known to induce atrial dysrhythmias, ventricular dysrhythmias, and overt ischemic changes on the ECG. These changes are often transient, as they were in this case—all signs of ischemia and the arrhythmia gradually resolved over the ensuing two hours. A cardiac catheterization was performed and demonstrated no significant coronary disease. Unfortunately the patient never regained normal neurologic function.

75. **Supraventricular tachycardia (SVT), rate 200.** The differential diagnosis of a regular narrow QRS complex tachycardia includes ST, atrial flutter, and SVT. ST can almost certainly be ruled out based on the rate of 200/min—the maximum sinus rate for most patients can be estimated as 220 – age; therefore, it is unlikely that this 60 year old woman could develop ST at a rate much greater than 160/minute. Evidence of atrial flutter is absent as well, leaving the diagnosis of SVT as the only possibility. Small retrograde P-waves can be seen just after the QRS complexes, a finding common in some types of SVT. Another common finding in SVTs is ST-segment depression, noted here in the inferior and lateral leads. This abnormality is sometimes inappropriately referred to as "rate-related ischemia." In fact, this ST-segment depression is not a reliable indicator of ischemia and does not reproduce during exercise testing. Its significance and etiology are uncertain.

This figure corresponds to case #75. Narrow QRS complex tachycardia consistent with supraventricular tachycardia

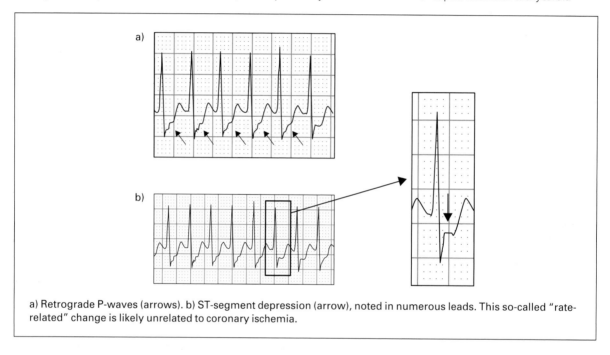

a) Retrograde P-waves (arrows). b) ST-segment depression (arrow), noted in numerous leads. This so-called "rate-related" change is likely unrelated to coronary ischemia.

76. **ST, rate 100, acute inferior-posterior-lateral MI.** STE with a convex upward morphology is present in the inferior and lateral leads, consistent with acute inferior-lateral MI. Tall R-waves, horizontal ST-segment depression, and upright T-waves in the right precordial leads are all strongly suggestive of acute posterior MI as well. Acute posterior MIs almost always occur in the presence of acute inferior MIs, although approximately 5% of the time they occur in isolation. The ST-segment depression noted in leads I and aVL represents reciprocal change from the acute MI. See figure opposite.

77. **SR, rate 60, acute anterior MI.** STE is present in leads V1–V4 consistent with acute MI. The morphology of the ST-segments is convex upwards in leads V2–V4, which might elicit some consideration of benign early repolarization (BER). However, the T-waves in these leads are abnormally large, especially in lead V3 (T-wave is larger than the QRS complex). This T-wave abnormality is often referred to as "hyperacute T-waves" which is suggestive of early acute cardiac ischemia. Two other findings exclude the diagnosis of BER: (1) the ST-segment in lead V1 is *convex* upwards; and (2) there is reciprocal ST-segment depression in the inferior leads. Additionally, lead aVL demonstrates an abnormal biphasic appearance of the T-wave, which suggests some lateral ischemia as well.

This figure corresponds to case #76

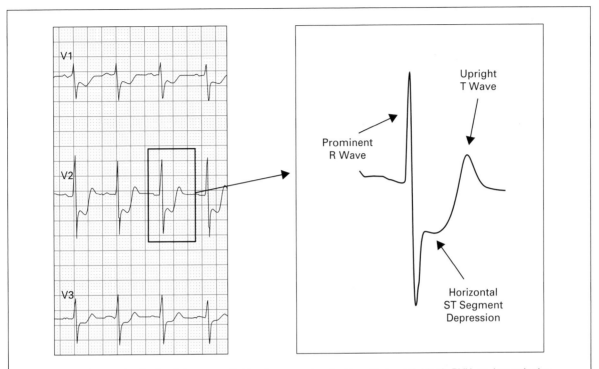

ST-segment depression in the right precordial leads, assuming that bundle branch block, RVH, and ventricular paced rhythms are not present, is suggestive of either anterior wall ischemia (non-infarction) or acute posterior wall STE MI. In patients with chest pain diagnosed with ACS, these two diagnoses occur in equal fashion. Horizontal or flat configuration of the ST-segment more strongly suggests acute posterior wall MI. The presence of a prominent R-wave and upright T-wave, along with horizontal ST-segment depression, is strongly suggestive of acute posterior wall MI as a cause of this ST-segment depression.

78. **AV junctional rhythm, rate 60, anteroseptal MI of undetermined age, inferolateral ischemia, consider LMCA occlusion.** This narrow QRS complex rhythm demonstrates no obvious P-waves and proceeds at a rate that is typical for an AV junctional pacing focus. Q-waves are noted in leads V1–V2 and poor R-wave progression is present (R-wave in lead V3 <3 mm), consistent with a anteroseptal MI of undetermined age. The presence of mild STE in leads V1 and V2 suggest that the MI is acute. Pronounced STE is present in leads aVR and aVL, and the STE in lead aVR is greater in magnitude than the STE in lead V1. Both of these findings are highly specific for coronary occlusion involving the LMCA (5,6). Involvement of the LMCA in ACS is associated with 70% mortality without prompt invasive therapy (percutaneous intervention, bypass surgery). See figure on p. 100.

79. **ST, rate 125, acute anterior-lateral MI.** At first glance, the ECG appears to be a wide QRS complex tachycardia. However, leads II and V1 clearly demonstrate that the QRS complexes are narrow, and it is the marked ST-segment deflections (elevations or depressions) that are giving the false appearance of wide QRS complexes. A *truly* wide QRS complex rhythm should demonstrate wide complexes in *all* of the leads. Marked STE is present in the anterior (V2–V4) and lateral (V5, V6, I, and aVL) leads, and reciprocal ST-segment depression is present in the inferior leads and in lead V1. When diffuse STE is present, these reciprocal changes exclude other causes of STE such as pericarditis, BER, ventricular aneurysm, and LVH.

This figure corresponds to case #78

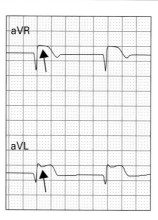

This electrocardiogram demonstrates significant abnormality and, thus, represents a high risk ECG. In particular, the presence of STE in leads aVR and aVL suggests a left main coronary artery occlusion. Furthermore, the STE in lead V1 as well as the widespread ST segment depression (leads II, III, aVF, V3 to V6) suggests a left main coronary artery occlusion.

80. **SR with first degree AV block, rate 83, acute anterior-lateral MI, possible inferior MI of undetermined age.** The PR-interval is 210 msec, diagnostic of a first degree AV block. Q-waves with STE are present in anterior leads V2–V4 and STE is also present in lateral leads I and aVL, consistent with an acute MI of the anterior and lateral walls.

81. **Atrial fibrillation, ventricular rate 130, aberrant ventricular conduction, suspected hyperkalemia.** The rhythm is slightly irregular and without obvious P-waves, suggestive of atrial fibrillation. The QRS complexes are wide, consistent with aberrant ventricular conduction. The marked QRS prolongation (200 msec) and sine-wave morphology of some leads is highly suggestive of hyperkalemia. The serum potassium in this case was 8.1 mEq/L (normal 3.5–5.1 mEq/L). Hyperkalemia is well-known to produce tachydysrhythmias, bradydysrhythmias, axis changes, ST-segment and T-wave changes, and conduction disturbances. See figure opposite.

82. **100% paced rhythm, rate 70.** Electronic pacer spikes precede each QRS complex. A leftward axis is present, typical of a right ventricular pacemaker site. Widening of the QRS complexes and "discordant" ST-segments are present, also typical of electronic pacemakers. Myocardial ischemia may be difficult to determine in the presence of an electronic pacemaker; however, loss of this discordant relationship between the QRS complexes and the ST-segments is a clue to the presence of ischemia. See figure opposite.

83. **ST, rate 125, left bundle branch block (LBBB).** A LBBB is diagnosed based on the presence of QRS widening >120 msec; broad monophasic R-waves in lateral leads I, V5, and V6; and rS complexes in the right precordial leads. The QRS complexes and ST-segments are appropriately "discordant" (leads in which the QRS complexes primarily point downward, e.g. leads V1–V3, demonstrate STE of up to 5 mm; and leads in which the QRS complexes primarily point upward, e.g. leads I, II, V6, demonstrate ST-segment depression of up to 5 mm). This "appropriate discordance" between the QRS complexes and ST-segments is normal in the setting of LBBB or right ventricular electronic pacemakers (see prior case). Loss of this discordant relationship, i.e. "concordance," is a highly specific marker of myocardial ischemia. See figure on p. 102.

This figure corresponds to case #81

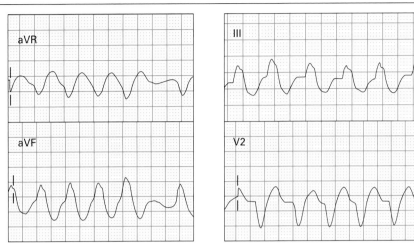

The markedly wide QRS complex rhythm of severe hyperkalemia is a pre-arrest rhythm. It is characterized by a very wide QRS complexes of variable rate. The P-waves are not present though the mechanism of the dysrhythmia is likely sinus in origin with premature complexes; in these instances, in the absence of obvious atrial beats, the rhythm must be diagnosed as atrial fibrillation. The "classic" sine-wave configuration (as seen in leads aVR and aVF) is very suggestive of hyperkalemia. Certain leads will demonstrate a wide QRS complex (as seen in leads III and V2) without apparent sine-wave configuration—this morphology is still strongly suggestive of an elevated serum potassium level yet difficult to distinguish from other widened QRS complex presentations.

This figure corresponds to case #82

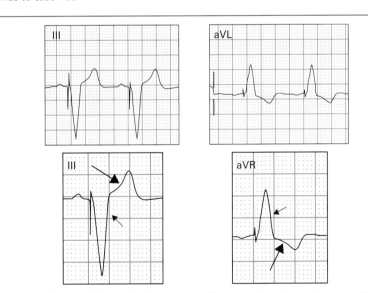

The right ventricular paced electrocardiographic rhythm markedly reduces the diagnostic power of the 12-lead ECG in the evaluation of the patient suspected of myocardial ischemia or infarction. The appropriate relationship of the QRS complex with the ST-segment/T-wave is referred to as "appropriate discordance." In this relationship, the major, terminal portion of the QRS complex is oriented on the opposite side of the isoelectric baseline from the ST-segment and T-wave. In lead III, the QRS complex (small arrow) is located opposite from the ST-segment/T-wave (large arrow)—in this case, demonstrating discordant STE. In lead aVR, the QRS complex (small arrow) is positive such that the ST-segment and T-wave (large arrow) are located on opposite sides of the electrical baseline—here, manifesting discordant ST-segment depression. Both of the electrocardiographic findings are the normal or expected ST-segment/T-wave configurations for the right ventricular paced electrocardiographic rhythm.

This figure corresponds to case #83

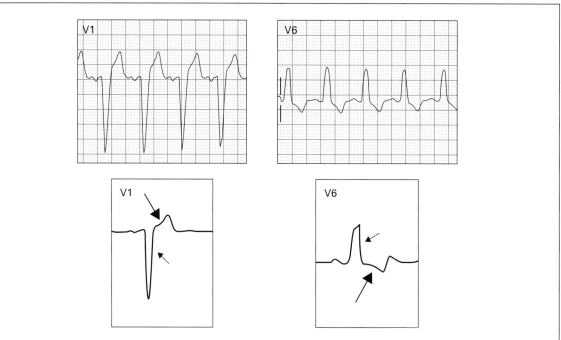

The LBBB pattern markedly reduces the diagnostic power of the 12-lead ECG in the evaluation of the patient suspected of ACS. The appropriate relationship of the QRS complex with the ST-segment/T-wave is referred to as "appropriate discordance." In this relationship, the major, terminal portion of the QRS complex is oriented on the opposite side of the isoelectric baseline from the ST-segment and T-wave. In lead V1, the QRS complex (small arrow) is located opposite from the ST-segment/T-wave (large arrow)—in this case, demonstrating discordant STE. In lead V6, the QRS complex (small arrow) is positive such that the ST-segment and T-wave (large arrow) are located on opposite sides of the electrical baseline—here, manifesting discordant ST-segment depression. Both of the electrocardiographic findings are the normal or expected ST-segment/T-wave configurations for the LBBB pattern.

84. **SR, rate 85, left ventricular hypertrophy (LVH) with repolarization changes.** LVH is diagnosed based on the amplitudes of the S-wave in lead V1 + R-wave in lead V6 >35 mm. LVH is often associated with asymmetric T-wave inversions in leads I, aVL, V4–V6 due to abnormal ventricular repolarization. Slight ST-segment depression may be present in these leads as well. This T-wave finding is often referred to simply as "LVH with repolarization abnormality" or "LVH with strain pattern." This abnormality does not represent acute myocardial ischemia. Less commonly, lead II may demonstrate this finding as well. The presence of T-wave inversions in any other limb or precordial leads or the presence of *symmetric* T-wave inversions should always be assumed to represent cardiac ischemia. LVH is often mistakenly misdiagnosed as myocardial ischemia, and vice-versa, because of these repolarization abnormalities. A comparison to prior ECGs is very helpful in distinguishing this normal variant from true myocardial ischemia.

85. **a) Atrial fibrillation, rate 160, probable WPW.** The rhythm is irregularly irregular with wide QRS complexes. The two main diagnostic considerations are atrial fibrillation with bundle branch block and atrial fibrillation with WPW. Although the major portion of the ECG shows only minor beat-to-beat variation, favoring a bundle branch block, the final quarter of the rhythm demonstrates much more variation in the QRS morphology and width. This is characteristic of the presence of an accessory pathway. There are two other findings that favor WPW versus a bundle branch block: (1) A tall R-wave is present in lead V1. This could be attributed to either RBBB or WPW.

However, RBBB should produce either a qR complex or an rsR' (taller "right rabbit ear") pattern, neither of which is present, thus excluding RBBB; (2) A leftward axis is present. Leftward axis is typical of either LBBB or WPW. However, there are no other major criteria that meet the definition of a LBBB (broad monophasic R-waves in leads V5–V6; rS waves in right precordial leads), therefore LBBB is excluded.

b) Atrial fibrillation, rate 150, WPW. The ECG was obtained during procainamide infusion. Procainamide is generally considered the best pharmacologic treatment (medications with AV-nodal blocking effects may facilitate conduction through the accessory pathway, resulting in increased ventricular rates and hemodynamic collapse). The ECG demonstrates the same diagnostic features noted in Figure a) below, and beat-to-beat variability typical of atrial fibrillation with WPW has become more pronounced.

c) SR, rate 77, WPW. The patient has converted to SR with procainamide infusion. The typical triad of WPW is present: shortened PR-interval (<120 msec), slightly widened QRS complex (≥100 msec), and delta-wave. Note that the delta-wave is only apparent in some, but not all, leads. Perhaps the most notable finding in patients with WPW is the presence of the shortened PR-interval, which generally is apparent in *all* leads. WPW often produces Q-waves in inferior leads with a leftward axis which may be misdiagnosed as a prior inferior MI. WPW also may produce a tall R-wave in lead V1 which may be misdiagnosed as a prior posterior MI. Both pseudo-infarction patterns are present in this case. See figure below.

This figure corresponds to case #85

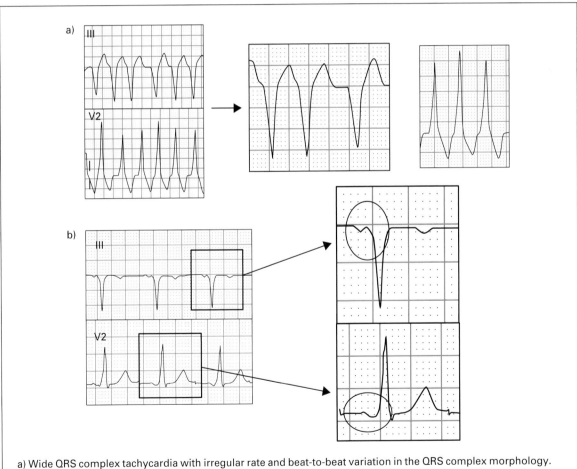

a) Wide QRS complex tachycardia with irregular rate and beat-to-beat variation in the QRS complex morphology. This dysrhythmia is atrial fibrillation in the setting of WPW. b) Note the classic triad of shortened PR-interval, widened QRS complex, and delta-wave. Note the negatively oriented delta-wave occurring in the Q wave in lead III.

86. **Accelerated idioventricular rhythm versus sinoventricular rhythm, rate 115, ventricular pause, suspected hyperkalemia.** A wide QRS complex tachycardia is present without obvious atrial activity, suggesting a primary ventricular rhythm. When the rate of a ventricular rhythm is between 40–120/minute, the rhythm is referred to as an accelerated idioventricular rhythm. The marked widening of the QRS complexes (200 msec) is unusual even for ventricular rhythms, however, and should call into consideration the possibility of a metabolic abnormality such as hyperkalemia or sodium-channel blocking drug toxicity. Both of these conditions are well-known to produce pseudo-ventricular rhythms with marked widening of QRS complexes, although hyperkalemia is the more likely of the two to produce unusual AV blocks and pauses on the rhythm (noted in the first half of the rhythm). Hyperkalemia preferentially affects atrial tissue and suppresses the appearance of P-waves, even when sinus node activity is still present and activating the ventricle. This is referred to as a "sinoventricular rhythm." When treatment is initiated, the P-waves seem to reappear. In reality, sinus activity was always present but simply not visible as P-waves. This patient did, in fact, have severe hyperkalemia. Administration of intravenous sodium bicarbonate and insulin resulted in the reappearance of P-waves and narrowing of the QRS complexes.

87. **SR, rate 83, peaked T-waves suggestive of hyperkalemia.** T-waves associated with hyperkalemia are typically abnormally large and, unlike other causes of prominent T-waves (acute myocardial ischemia, acute pericarditis, LVH, BER, bundle branch block, and pre-excitation syndromes), they tend to be peaked and narrow-based. Peaked T-waves are generally the earliest ECG finding in the presence of hyperkalemia. Their appearance does not correlate with specific serum potassium levels. With progression of hyperkalemia, other ECG abnormalities develop including P-wave flattening, PR-interval and QRS prolongation, high-grade AV blocks, intraventricular conduction abnormalities (including fascicular blocks and bundle branch blocks), and finally a sine-wave appearance on the rhythm. This patient's serum potassium level was 7.1 mEq/L (normal 3.5–5.3 mEq/L). See figure below.

This figure corresponds to case #87. The prominent T-waves of hyperkalemia

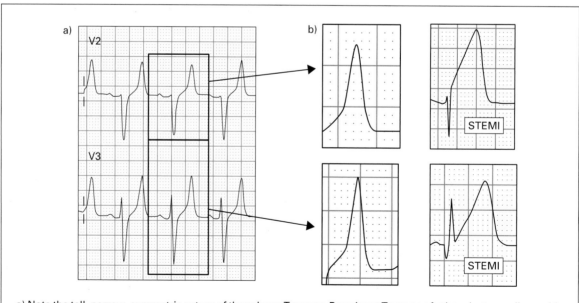

a) Note the tall, narrow, symmetric nature of these large T-waves. Prominent T-waves of other electrocardiographic entities, such as early acute MI, are wide-based, less tall, and asymmetric. b) Prominent T-waves of early ischemia are wide-based and asymmetric.

88. **SVT, rate 130.** A regular, narrow QRS complex tachycardia is present. The differential diagnosis in this setting includes ST, atrial flutter, and SVT. Regular sinus activity is absent, and evidence of atrial flutter is also absent. Small retrograde P-waves are present immediately following the QRS complexes in the inferior leads as well as lead V1. This is a common finding with SVTs.

89. **ST, rate 150, left posterior fascicular block (LPFB), lateral ischemia.** a) The 12-lead ECG in Figure a) (p. 63) demonstrates a regular, narrow QRS complex tachycardia. As noted in the prior case, the main diagnostic considerations are ST, atrial flutter, and SVT. Close scrutiny of all leads reveals evidence of P-waves in the precordial leads which cause an upward deflection on the terminal portion of the T-waves, consistent with ST. A rightward axis is present as well. The differential diagnosis for rightward axis includes LPFB, prior lateral MI, right ventricular hypertrophy, acute (e.g. pulmonary embolism) or chronic (e.g. emphysema) lung disease, ventricular ectopy, hyperkalemia, overdoses of sodium-channel blocking drugs, and misplaced limb leads. This ECG meets criteria for LPFB based on rightward axis, rS complexes in leads I and aVL and qR complexes in lead III. Slight ST-segment depression is present in the lateral leads suggesting lateral ischemia.
b) The rhythm strip was obtained at rapid chart speed (50 mm/sec). Performance of the ECG or rhythm strip at this speed "stretches out" the complexes and allows more clear delineation of the atrial and ventricular activity. This is particularly helpful at unmasking flutter waves that may be "hidden" within T-waves on the standard 12-lead ECG. In this case, the sinus node activity becomes more obvious, and absence of flutter waves is confirmed.

90. **a) SR, rate 71, poor R-wave progression, inferior and anterolateral ischemia, consider Wellens' syndrome.** T-wave inversions are present in the inferior and anterior leads consistent with diffuse ischemia. The deep symmetric appearance of the T-waves in the anterior leads is suggestive of Wellens' syndrome, an indication of critical stenosis in the proximal LAD artery (see case #38 for more detailed description). Poor R-wave progression, diagnosed based on R-wave amplitude in lead V3 <3 mm, is present and suggestive of a prior anteroseptal MI.
b) ST, rate 105, acute anterior-lateral MI. Wellens and colleagues[4] originally described that 75% of their patients with the T-wave abnormality developed extensive anterior MI within weeks if managed without invasive therapy. This patient did, in fact, develop an acute MI within days. Q-waves are present in leads V1, V2, I, and aVL; and STE is present in leads V1–V4 as well as leads I and aVL consistent with acute MI of the anterior and lateral walls. The infarct-related artery in this case was the LAD, as expected based on the ECG from 2 days earlier shown in Figure a). See figure on p. 106.

91. **AV junctional rhythm, rate 42.** A bradycardic rhythm without obvious P-waves is noted. The QRS complex is narrow, excluding a ventricular escape rhythm. The narrow QRS complexes and the rate (40–60/minute) is typical of an AV junctional rhythm.

92. **a) Probable ST, rate 113, rightward axis, non-specific intraventricular conduction delay, prolonged QT-interval, consider sodium-channel blocking drug toxicity or overdose.** P-waves are difficult to find, although some leads demonstrate subtle upward deflections on the terminal portions of the T-waves, suggesting atrial activity. A rightward axis is present, the differential diagnosis of which includes LPFB, prior lateral MI, right ventricular hypertrophy, acute (e.g. pulmonary embolism) or chronic (e.g. emphysema) lung disease, ventricular ectopy, hyperkalemia, overdoses of sodium-channel blocking drugs, and misplaced limb leads. Of these possibilities, only sodium-channel blocking drug toxicity would account for the non-specific intraventricular conduction delay (QRS duration 120 msec) and the prolonged QT-interval (QT = 400 msec, QTc = 550 msec). One additional finding that favors sodium-channel blocking drug toxicity is the presence of a prominent R'-wave in lead aVR.
b) WCT, rate 130. In the absence of any other history or the prior ECG, VT must be diagnosed based on the presence of a regular, wide QRS complex tachycardia with a rate >120/minute and absence of P-waves. The QRS complexes, however, are markedly wide (>200 msec) even for a ventricular rhythm, which should elicit

This figure corresponds to case #90

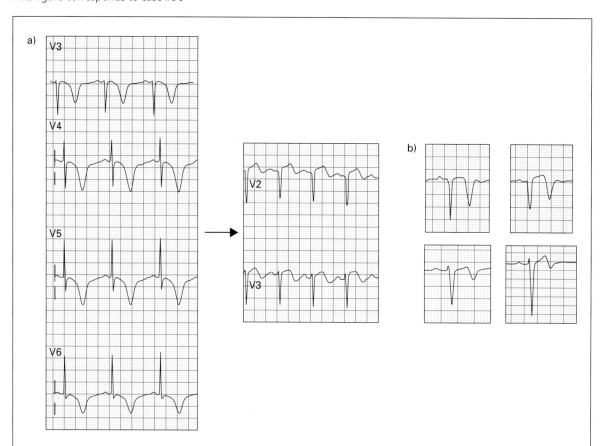

a) The deeply inverted, symmetric T-wave abnormalities seen in this example are a manifestation of Wellens' syndrome. Wellens' syndrome classically describes patients presenting without active chest pain and who lack cardiac biomarker abnormalities of myocardial infarction but demonstrate very specific T-wave abnormalities which have been found to signify underlying critical stenosis of the proximal LAD artery. The natural history of this syndrome is anterior wall MI within weeks if the patients are not treated invasively (i.e. with PCI), as occurred here, due to LAD occlusion. b) Two types of T-wave inversion have been described in Wellens' syndrome, including the deeply inverted, symmetric T-wave (upper) and the biphasic T-wave (lower).

consideration of a metabolic abnormality such as hyperkalemia or sodium-channel blocking drug toxicity. Both of these conditions are well-known to produce pseudo-ventricular rhythms with marked widening of QRS complexes that may sometimes seem bizarre in appearance. Both conditions also tend to suppress the appearance of P-waves on the ECG. Distinction between hyperkalemia versus sodium-channel blocking drug toxicity is very difficult when faced with a wide QRS complex tachycardia such as in this case (especially in the absence of historical information). Fortunately, treatment of either condition with intravenous sodium bicarbonate is effective treatment and produces reappearance of the P-waves, narrowing of the QRS complexes, and slowing of the ventricular rate at which point the presence or absence of peaked T-waves reveals the diagnosis. In this case, the patient received intravenous sodium bicarbonate with all of these improvements, indicating that the rhythm was actually just sinus tachycardia with aberrant conduction rather than VT. The T-waves remained normal in appearance, confirming the diagnosis of sodium-channel blocking drug toxicity. See figure opposite.

This figure corresponds to case #92

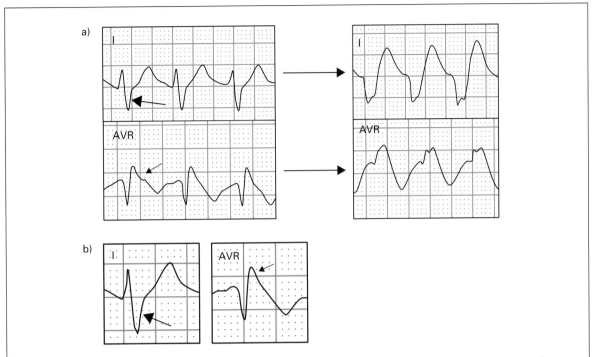

a) One of the causes of wide QRS complex tachycardia is sodium-channel blockade, in this case due to tricyclic antidepressant poisoning. Note the rapid rate (110–130/minute), widened QRS complexes, and prominent S-waves (large arrow) in lead I and prominent R' wave (small arrow) in lead aVR. Note also the progression of the syndrome with progressive widening of the QRS complex over approximately 30 minutes. b) Deep S-wave in lead I (large arrow), R' wave in lead aVR (small arrow), consistent with rightward deviation of the terminal QRS complex in a patient with TCA poisoning. Sinus tachycardia with a minimally widened QRS complex is also suggestive of TCA poisoning.

93. **a) Atrial fibrillation, rate 138, occasional aberrant conduction, acute inferior-lateral and probable posterior MI.** Although there appear to be occasional P-waves, the rhythm overall is irregularly irregular without consistent evidence of atrial activity, typical of atrial fibrillation. New-onset atrial fibrillation often produces atrial waves that give a false appearance of organized atrial activity. Occasional wide QRS complexes are present with a right bundle branch block morphology (aberrant conduction). Occasional aberrant conduction is common in atrial fibrillation. ST-segment elevation consistent with acute MI is present in the inferior and lateral leads. Pronounced ST-segment depression with relatively large R-waves is present in the right precordial leads, suggestive of posterior wall extension of the acute MI.

   b) Acute posterior MI. Posterior leads V8 and V9, placed on the left mid-back area just below the tip of the scapula, demonstrate STE confirming acute posterior MI. The right-sided lead RV4, placed on the right anterior chest wall, does *not* demonstrate STE, thereby excluding right ventricular MI. See figure on p. 108.

94. **SR with first degree AV block, rate 100, frequent premature AV junctional complexes, bifascicular block (RBBB + LAFB), acute anterior MI.** The majority of QRS complexes are preceded by P-waves with a prolonged PR-interval (first degree AV block). Frequent premature complexes are present with a morphology that is

This figure corresponds to case #93

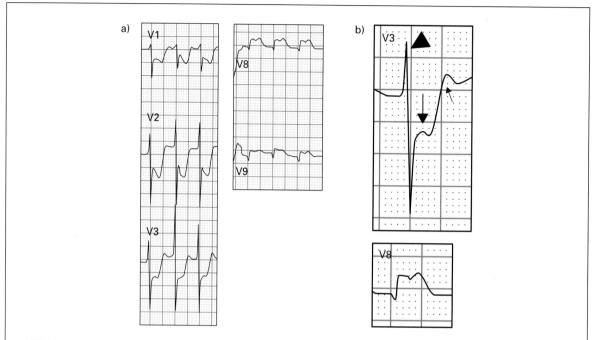

a) Right to mid precordial leads (V1 to V3) demonstrating significant ST-segment depression with prominent R-wave and upright T-wave, indicative of acute posterior wall MI. Leads V8 and V9, placed on the patient's left back, demonstrate STE, consistent with acute posterior wall MI. The inferior and lateral walls also demonstrate STE—this is a rather large myocardial infarction with three walls of the left ventricle affected. b) Lead V3 demonstrating significant ST-segment depression (large arrow) with prominent R-wave (arrowhead) and upright T-wave (small arrow), indicative of acute posterior wall MI. Lead V8 demonstrating STE, consistent with acute posterior wall MI.

identical to the underlying rhythm, suggesting that these are supraventricular in origin rather than PVCs. Absence of P-waves preceding these complexes suggests that they are originating in the AV junction. A RBBB is present as well as LAFB (leftward axis, rS complexes in lead III, qR complexes in I and aVL). STE is present in the anterior leads consistent with acute MI. See figure opposite.

95. **SR with first degree AV block, rate 83, bifascicular block (RBBB + LAFB).** This ECG is similar to the one in the preceding case in terms of the conduction block, but evidence of acute ischemia is lacking in this case. In the presence of a normal RBBB, the ST-segments should remain isoelectric. Slight ST-segment depression and T-wave inversions is permitted in the right precordial leads only, but ST-segment depression or T-wave inversions in any other leads or any STE should always be considered abnormal. See figure opposite.

96. **SB with first degree AV block, rate 43, acute inferior-lateral and probable posterior MI.** STE is present in leads II, III, aVF, and V5-V6, consistent with acute inferior-lateral MI. Q-waves are beginning to form in leads III and aVF as well, producing the leftward axis. Reciprocal ST-segment depression is present in leads I and aVL. ST-segment depression is also present in leads V1–V4, which may represent reciprocal change or posterior extension of the MI. The presence of tall R-waves with horizontal ST-segment depression in these leads favors posterior MI. The diagnosis was confirmed by noting STE in posteriorly placed leads. See figure on p. 110.

This figure corresponds to case #94. RBBB with acute anterior wall MI

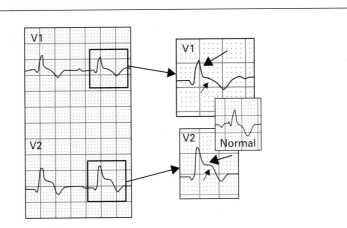

Leads V1–V3 in patients with RBBB are similar to those of patients with LBBB and ventricular paced rhythm patterns in that the major, terminal portion of the QRS complex is often located on the opposite side of the baseline from the ST-segment/T-wave complex. In this example, the ST-segment (small arrow) is located on the same side of the baseline as the primary, terminal portion of the QRS complex (large arrow)—demonstrating concordant STE. The insert demonstrates the normal relationship of the ST-segment to the major, terminal portion of the QRS complex.

This figure corresponds to case #95

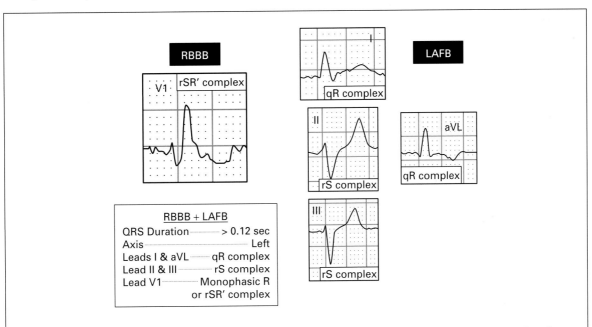

This bifascicular block, RBBB plus LAFB, is detected on the ECG when RBBB is noted with a leftward axis. Recall that a normal axis is usually seen in RBBB. Further analysis demonstrates a qR complex in leads I and aVL as well as an rS complex in leads II and III—these findings, in conjunction with leftward axis, account for the LAFB.

This figure corresponds to case #96

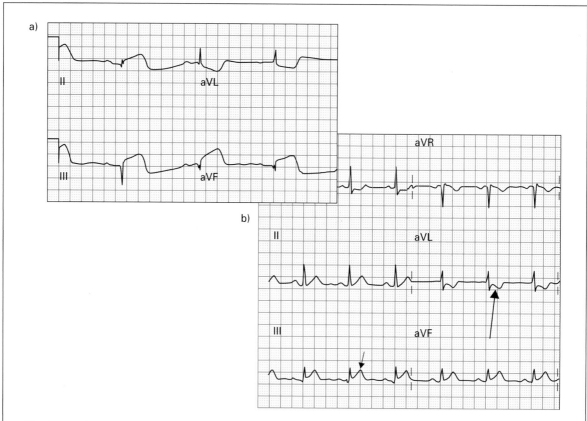

a) Reciprocal ST-segment depression, colloquially referred to as "reciprocal change," is defined as ST-segment depression on the ECG of a patient with STE simultaneously occurring elsewhere on that same electrocardiogram. This form of ST-segment depression is of value for two reasons: (1) its presence provides very convincing electrocardiographic evidence that the STE results from acute MI; and (2) it identifies a patient at increased cardiovascular risk as a result of the acute MI. One caveat should be kept in mind, however: ST-segment depression is a normal finding in some cases (e.g. LBBB, RBBB, paced rhythms, and ventricular hypertrophy) and should not be considered reciprocal change. b) In instances of subtle STE (small arrow), the reciprocal change in lead aVL (large arrow) strongly supports the diagnosis of acute inferior MI.

97.   **SR, rate 93, acute pericarditis.** Slight STE is noted in several leads, most notably leads V2–V4. In a young patient, the main considerations in this setting might be BER, acute pericarditis, and to a lesser extent acute MI. However, subtle PR-segment depression is present especially in leads II and aVF; and subtle PR-segment elevation is present in lead aVR, strongly suggesting acute pericarditis as the diagnosis. See figure opposite.

98.   **SR, rate 71, BER.** STE is present in multiple leads. The differential diagnosis for diffuse STE includes large MI, acute pericarditis, BER, LVH, and coronary vasospasm. The patient's age and the notching of the J-point in leads V4–V5 is typical of BER, though not completely diagnostic. Serial ECGs were performed and demonstrated no evolving changes of acute MI. The use of serial ECGs can be very helpful in distinguishing acute MI versus BER and other benign causes of STE. Acute MI will usually demonstrate evolving changes in the ST-segments and/or T-waves during serial performance of the ECGs. See figure opposite.

This figure corresponds to case #97

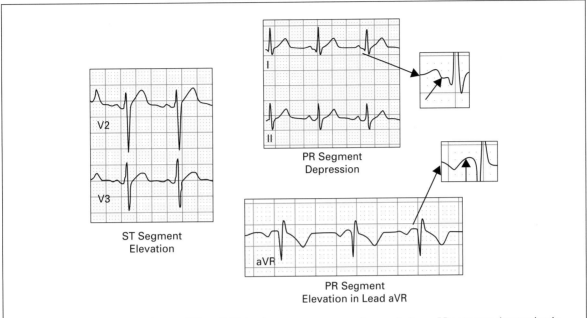

ST Segment
Elevation

PR Segment
Depression

PR Segment
Elevation in Lead aVR

Acute pericarditis can manifest as diffuse STE that has a convex upwards morphology. PR segment depression in those leads with STE, and PR segment elevation in lead aVR, are common as well. When the myocardium is also involved, referred to as acute *myopericarditis*, the STE can manifest electrocardiographically by STE of various forms (convex, concave, and obliquely straight).

This figure corresponds to case #98

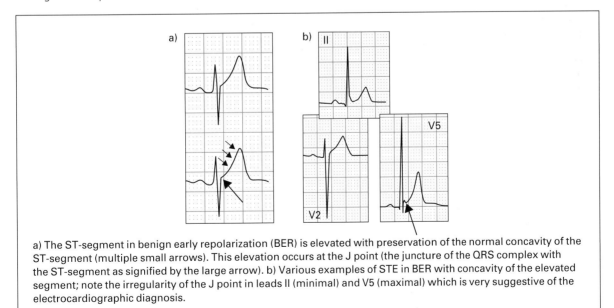

a) The ST-segment in benign early repolarization (BER) is elevated with preservation of the normal concavity of the ST-segment (multiple small arrows). This elevation occurs at the J point (the juncture of the QRS complex with the ST-segment as signified by the large arrow). b) Various examples of STE in BER with concavity of the elevated segment; note the irregularity of the J point in leads II (minimal) and V5 (maximal) which is very suggestive of the electrocardiographic diagnosis.

99. **a) SR, rate 88, acute inferior and possible posterior MI, lateral ischemia.** STE is present in the inferior leads consistent with acute MI. ST-depression with upright T-waves is present in the right precordial leads suggestive of acute posterior MI, although tall R-waves have not yet developed which would more strongly favor this diagnosis. T-wave inversions and ST-segment depression consistent with ischemia is present in the lateral leads.

b) A 15-lead ECG is shown, demonstrating the standard 12 leads plus a right precordial lead (lead V7) to evaluate right ventricular involvement and two posterior leads (leads V8–V9) to evaluate posterior involvement. In this case, the extra leads do not appear to demonstrate any right ventricular or posterior infarction.

c) An 80-lead ECG is shown (single complexes presented). Detailed instruction in interpretation of this ECG is beyond the scope of this text, but to summarize the findings: leads 5–7 are right precordial leads, and they demonstrate slight STE, consistent with right ventricular MI; leads 72–77 are posterior thorax leads, and they also demonstrate slight STE consistent with posterior MI. The increased information from this technology allows us to diagnose evidence of acute posterior and right ventricular MI even when the 15-lead ECG appeared to demonstrate an isolated inferior MI.

d) The figure demonstrates body surface mapping with torso imaging. The blue area on the anterior thorax (left) indicates ST-segment depression and the red area on the posterior thorax (right) indicates STE.

100. **SR, rate 86.** Aside from the artifact, the ECG is normal. The sinus rhythm is diagnosed based on upright P-waves in all of the limb leads with the exception of lead aVR, in which sinus P-waves are expected to be inverted; and there is a 1:1 relationship between P-waves and QRS complexes. All intervals are normal, the axis is normal, and there are no ST-segment elevations or depressions. T-wave inversions are normally found in lead aVR and often in V1. Despite the normalcy of this ECG, the patient was diagnosed with acute MI based on positive cardiac biomarkers. ST-segment and T-wave changes later developed with persistence of pain. In the presence of acute myocardial ischemia or infarction the initial ECG is diagnostic in only approximately 50% of patients. Acquisition of serial ECGs can significantly increase the yield, but a completely normal ECG may still remain and should not be used in isolation to exclude the diagnosis of acute ischemia or infarction.

101. **SR, rate 93, LBBB.** A wide QRS complex rhythm is present. Causes of QRS complex widening (QRS duration >100 msec) include hypothermia, hyperkalemia, aberrant intraventricular conduction (e.g. bundle branch block), ventricular ectopy, electronic pacemakers, medications (extensive list, but typical for those that block sodium channels), and LVH. When the cause of QRS complex widening is not identified from this list, the term "non-specific intraventricular conduction delay" is often used. Other abnormalities noted in the ECG include leftward axis (differential diagnosis includes LAFB, LBBB, prior inferior MI, LVH, ventricular ectopy, electronic pacemakers, and WPW), and discordance between the QRS complexes and the ST-segments. These findings are all typical characteristics of an uncomplicated LBBB. The diagnostic criteria for LBBB also includes the presence of rS complexes in the right precordial leads and broad monophasic R waves in leads I, V5, and V6. The diagnosis of a full bundle branch block requires the QRS duration ≥120 msec. If all criteria are met but the duration of the QRS is <120 msec, an "incomplete" bundle branch block is diagnosed.

102. **SR, rate 90, occasional aberrantly conducted complexes, inferior-posterior-anterior MI of undetermined age, non-specific T-wave flattening diffusely.** Significant size Q-waves are present in the inferior leads consistent with inferior MI. The absence of ST-segment changes *suggests* that infarction is not ongoing, but rather of indeterminate age. Similarly, precordial leads V4–V6 demonstrate small q-waves, and of greater concern is the loss or normal R-waves in leads V3–V4. ST-segment abnormalities are absent. These findings strongly suggest anterolateral MI of undetermined age. A relatively tall R-wave (defined as R:S ratio ≥1) is present in lead V1. The differential diagnosis of a tall R-wave in lead V1 includes WPW, posterior MI, RBBB (or incomplete RBBB), ventricular ectopy, right ventricular hypertrophy, acute right ventricular dilatation (right ventricular "strain," e.g.

This figure corresponds to case #102

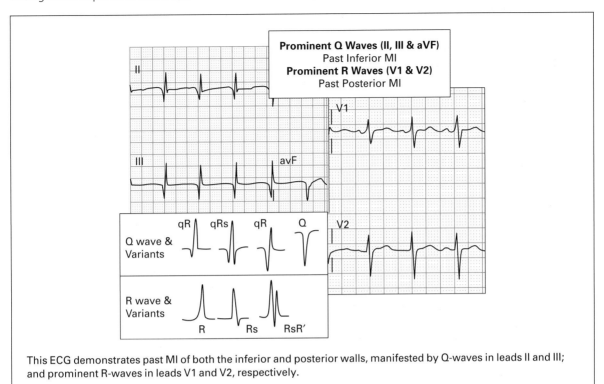

Prominent Q Waves (II, III & aVF)
Past Inferior MI
Prominent R Waves (V1 & V2)
Past Posterior MI

Q wave & Variants
qR   qRs   qR   Q

R wave & Variants
R   Rs   RsR′

This ECG demonstrates past MI of both the inferior and posterior walls, manifested by Q-waves in leads II and III; and prominent R-waves in leads V1 and V2, respectively.

massive pulmonary embolism), hypertrophic cardiomyopathy, progressive muscular dystrophy, dextrocardia, and misplaced precordial leads. The evidence of a prior MI favors posterior MI as the likely cause of the tall R-wave in lead V1. Once prior ECGs were obtained for comparison, it was determined that all of the abnormalities on this patient's current ECG were unchanged and the result of a prior large MI. The 5th QRS complex on the ECG has a different morphology, likely the result of aberrant ventricular conduction. See figure above.

103. **SR, rate 68, BER.** Diffuse STE is present. The differential diagnosis of diffuse STE includes large MI, acute pericarditis, BER, LVH, and coronary vasospasm. The morphology of the STE is concave upwards and there are no reciprocal ST-segment depressions anywhere, favoring a non-ischemia diagnosis. PR-segment depression that is typical of acute pericarditis is absent. Very prominent T-waves with maximal STE in leads V2–V3 is present and is typical of BER. Nevertheless, when doubt exists as to the possibility of acute MI versus a benign cause of STE, acquisition of serial ECGs (or prior ECGs) for comparison is prudent. Benign causes of STE are expected to be static with time, whereas acute MI will likely demonstrate evolving ST-segment and T-wave changes.

104. **SR, rate 60, acute pericarditis.** STE is present in the precordial leads as well as lead II. Causes of diffuse STE can include large MIs, acute pericarditis, BER, LVH, and coronary vasospasm. Mild PR-segment depression is present in many of these leads, and mild PR-segment elevation is present in lead aVR, both of which strongly favor acute pericarditis amongst these causes.

105. **SR, rate 70, PRWP.** Sinus rhythm is diagnosed based on the presence of upright P-waves in all limb leads except for aVR, which has the expected inverted P-waves of sinus beats. All intervals are normal, a key finding in the presence of an overdose: many psychiatry medications have sodium-channel blocking effects, which would be expected to produce widening of the QRS complex and a prolonged QT-interval when taken in overdose; many cardiac medications produce bradycardia and AV blocks when taken in overdose. PRWP is diagnosed based on the R-wave in lead V3 <3 mm. PRWP may be a normal variant in young patients, although in older patients and patients with cardiac risk factors it suggests an anteroseptal MI of undetermined age.

106. **VT versus hyperkalemia, rate 150.** A wide QRS complex tachycardia is present without distinct atrial complexes. The QRS complexes are so wide (>200 msec) that hyperkalemia should be a strong consideration. Further favoring hyperkalemia as the diagnosis, the overall rhythm appears to be taking on a sine-wave pattern. The patient did, in fact, prove to have severe hyperkalemia (serum level 9.1 mEq/L; normal 3.5–5.3 mEq/L).

107. **SR, rate 88, LVH with repolarization abnormality.** LVH is diagnosed based on the amplitude of the S-wave in lead V1 + the amplitude of the R-wave in lead V5 (can use the larger R-wave between V5 or V6 for this calculation) >35 mm. Moderate to severe LVH often produces changes in ventricular depolarization and repolarization: the QRS may be slightly prolonged (though normal in this case), there may be slight J-point elevation in the right precordial leads and slight ST-segment depression in V4–V6, and asymmetric T-wave inversions may be present in the lateral leads I, aVL, V4–V6, and sometimes also in lead II. The T-wave (repolarization) abnormality is sometimes referred to as a "strain pattern." ST-segment or T-wave changes in other leads than those noted above should be assumed to represent myocardial ischemia until proven otherwise. See figure below.

This figure corresponds to case #107. The electrocardiographic findings of LVH

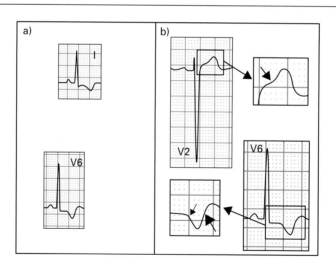

As noted, the LVH pattern is noted when the ECG demonstrates prominent QRS complexes in the precordial leads. Approximately 70% of these electrocardiographic LVH patterns will demonstrate ST-segment and/or T-wave abnormalities—the so-called "strain" pattern. a) Leads I and V6 demonstrating the strain pattern in LVH. b) Lead V2 demonstrates STE which is concave upward (arrow). Lead V6 with ST-segment depression and T-wave inversion; note the gradual downsloping of the initial limb (small arrow) of the ST/T complex and the more abrupt return to the baseline (large arrow) in its terminal form.

108. **a) SB, rate 46, anteroseptal ischemia versus early isolated acute posterior MI.** Slight ST-segment depression is present in the right precordial leads. This could represent acute myocardial ischemia or it could be the early phase of an isolated posterior MI. Posterior MI usually occurs in the presence of an inferior wall MI, but 5% will occur in isolation. The upright tall T-waves in the right precordial leads favors posterior MI; in the setting of just ischemia, the T-waves would be expected to be much smaller, flat, or inverted.

    b) Posterior leads demonstrate STE consistent with acute posterior MI. This case nicely illustrates the importance of posterior leads in patients with anteroseptal lead ST-segment depression. The finding of acute posterior MI via posterior leads qualifies this patient for emergent reperfusion therapy (fibrinolytics or PCI), whereas the standard 12-lead would suggest that this patient warrants only anti-ischemia therapy.

109. **SR, rate 75, acute inferior MI.** Subtle STE is present in the inferior leads consistent with an acute MI. The oblique (straight) morphology of the initial portion of the T-wave is an important clue to early ischemia. Reciprocal ST-segment depression is found in lateral leads I, aVL, V5, and V6. Lead aVF is an important lead in that it is probably the most sensitive lead for demonstrating reciprocal changes (usually T-wave inversion first, then ST-segment depression) in the presence of an acute inferior MI, and in fact these reciprocal changes in lead aVF may *precede* any ST-segment changes in the inferior leads.

110. **SB, rate 55, WPW.** P-waves are noted preceding each QRS complex, but the PR-interval is short (<120 msec). A short PR-interval should prompt consideration of WPW (the other most common cause of a short PR-interval is an AV junctional rhythm). This ECG does, in fact, demonstrate the classic triad of WPW: (1) short PR-interval, (2) delta-wave, and (3) slight prolongation of the QRS complex (≥100 msec). A leftward axis is present, common with WPW. Additionally, Q-waves are noted in inferior leads III and aVF. This pseudo-inferior MI appearance is a common finding reflecting abnormal depolarization in WPW; it is *not* an indication of a prior MI. WPW is also known to produce a pseudo-posterior MI appearance because of large R-waves in the right precordial leads.

References

1.   Marriott HJL. *Pearls and Pitfalls in Electrocardiography*, 2nd edn. Baltimore, MD: Williams & Wilkins, 1998.
2.   Hayden GE, Brady WJ, Perron AD, *et al.* Electrocardiographic T-wave inversion: differential diagnosis in the chest pain patient. *Am J Emerg Med* 2002;**20**:252–62.
3.   Kosuge M, Kimura K, Ishikawa T, *et al.* Electrocardiographic differentiation between acute pulmonary embolism and acute coronary syndromes on the basis of negative T waves. *Am J Cardiol* 2007;**99**:817–21.
4.   De Zwann C, Bar FW, Wellens HJJ. Characteristic electrocardiographic pattern indicating a critical stenosis high in left anterior descending coronary artery in patients admitted because of impending myocardial infarction. *Am Heart J* 1982;**103**:730–6.
5.   Kurisu S, Inoue I, Kawagoe T, *et al.* Electrocardiographic features in patients with acute myocardial infarction associated with left main coronary artery occlusion. *Heart* 2004;**90**:1059–60.
6.   Yamaji H, Iwasaki K, Kusachi S, *et al.* Prediction of acute left main coronary artery obstruction by 12-lead electrocardiography. *J Am Coll Cardiol* 2001;**38**:1348–54.

Part 3

12-Lead ECGs (advanced level)

Case histories

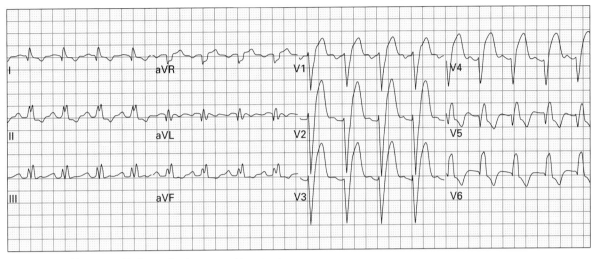

111. 67 year old woman with chest pain, dyspnea, and hypotension

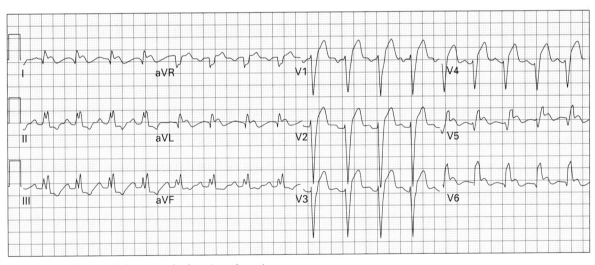

112. 42 year old man with chest pain, diaphoresis, and emesis

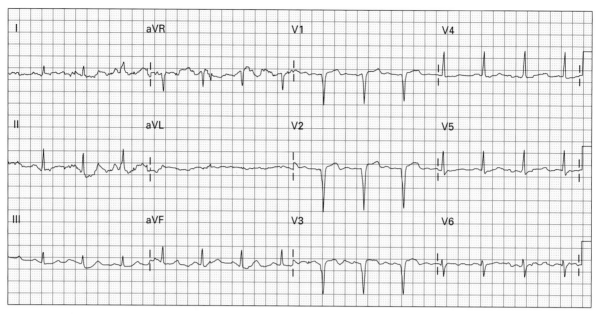

113. 67 year old woman with past MI and congestive heart failure presents with recurrent chest pain

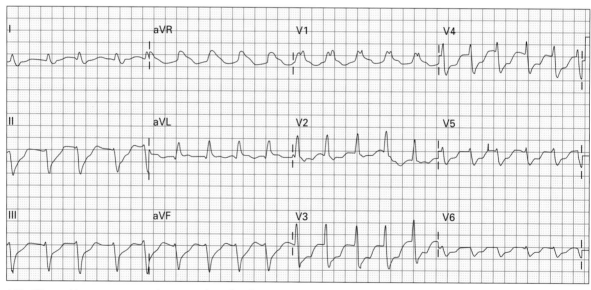

114. 22 year old woman presents after an overdose of medications

a)

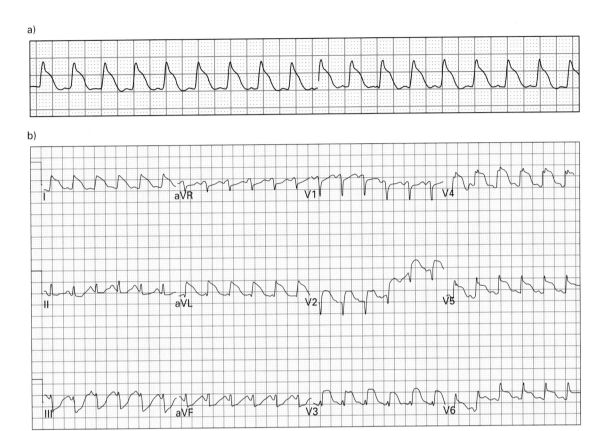

b)

115. a) and b) 58 year old woman with chest pain, hypotension, and pulmonary congestion

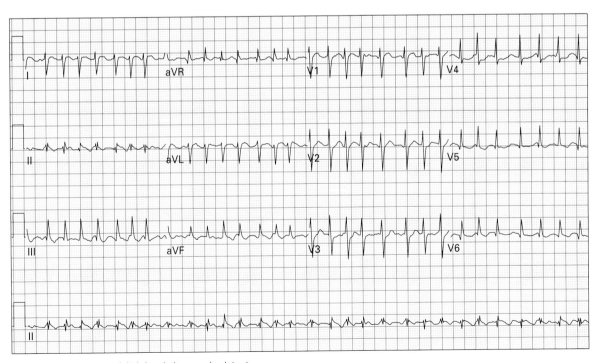

116. 61 year old man with lightheadedness and palpitations

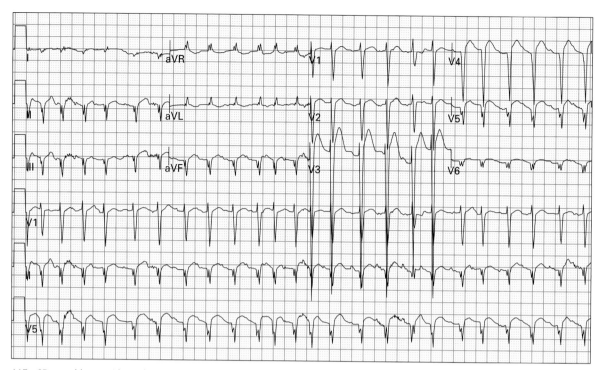

117. 65 year old man with emphysema presents with dyspnea and chest tightness

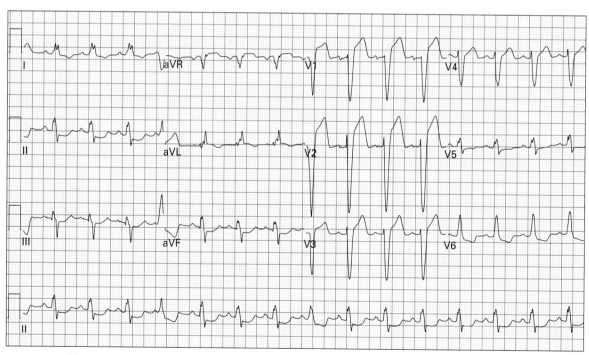

118. 66 year old man with left shoulder pain and dyspnea

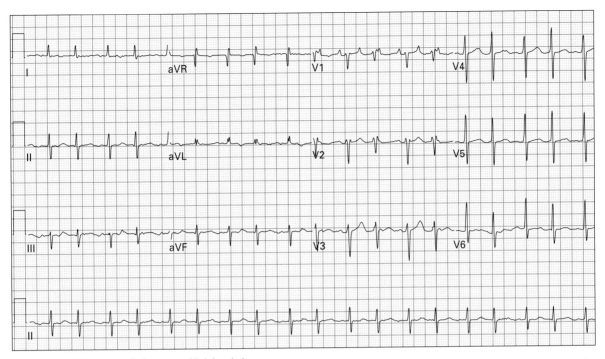

119. 54 year old woman with dyspnea and lightheadedness

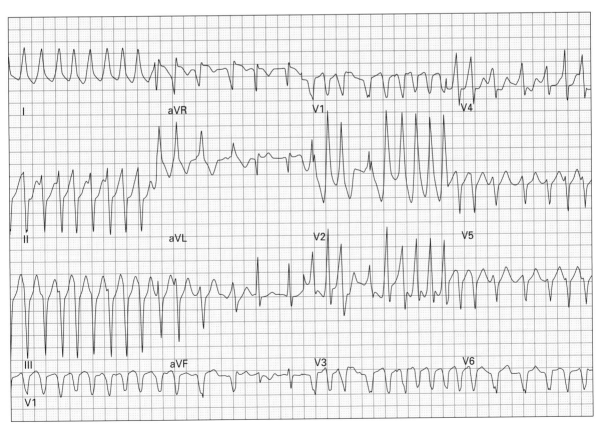

120. 26 year old man with dyspnea and palpitations

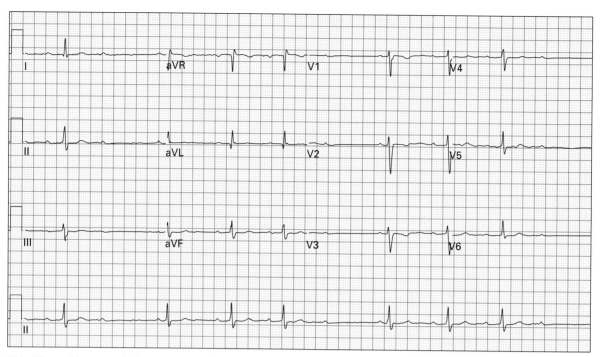

121. 33 year old woman who is asymptomatic; the ECG was obtained because she was noted to have a slow pulse

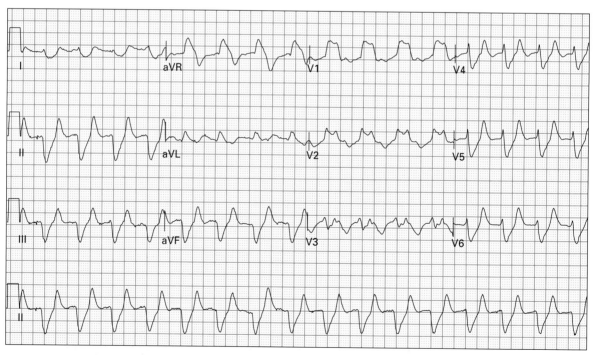

122. 55 year old man with history of renal failure presents obtunded

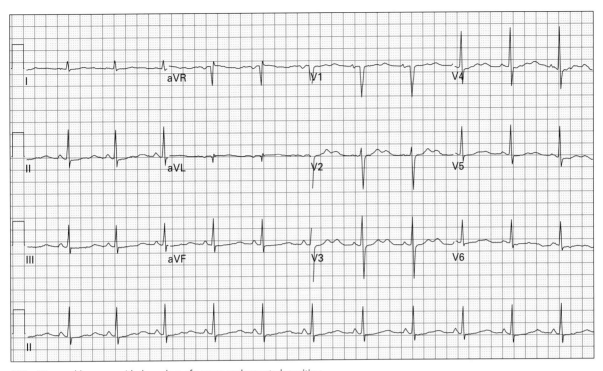

123. 47 year old woman with three days of nausea and repeated vomiting

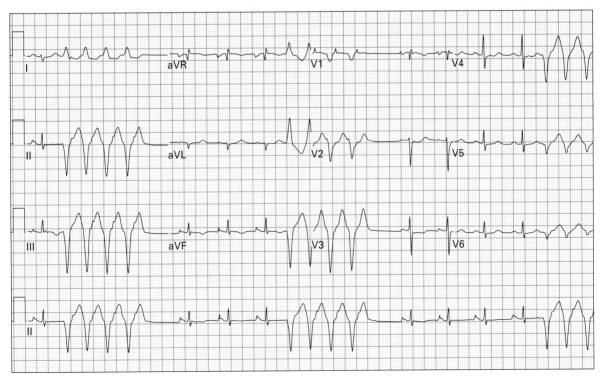

124. 42 year old woman with chest pain and dyspnea

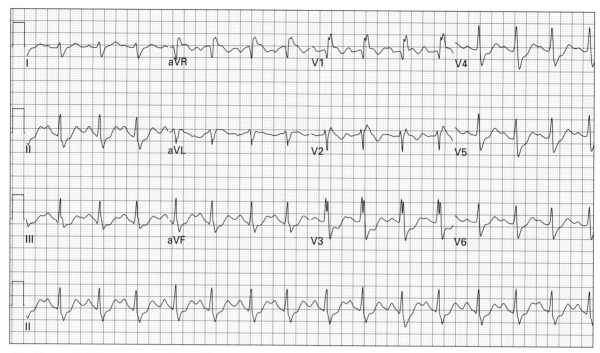

125. 15 year old girl presents unconscious and hypotensive; no other history is available

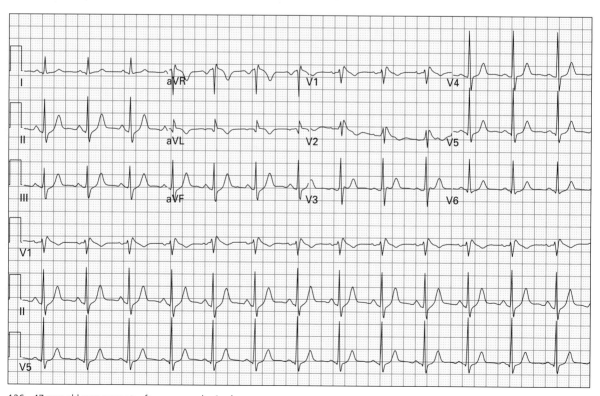

126. 47 year old man presents after a syncopal episode

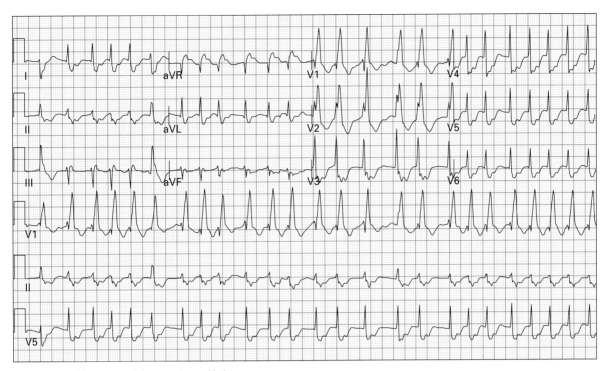

127. 66 year old woman with hypotension and lethargy

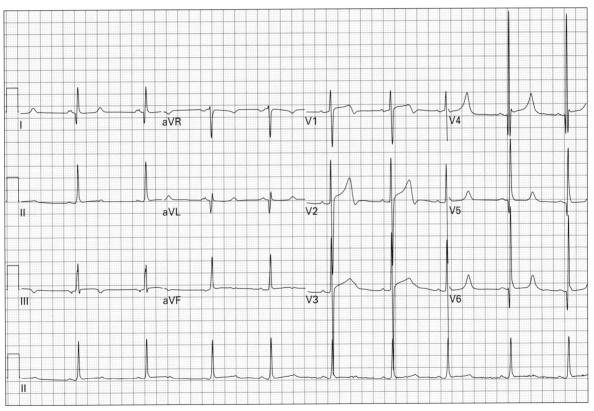

128. 29 year old man presents after a syncopal episode

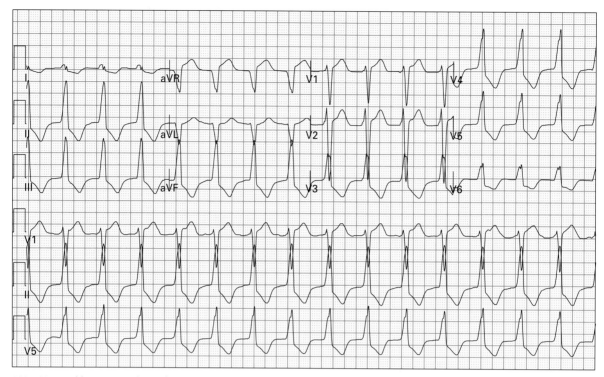

129. 68 year old woman one hour after receiving fibrinolytics for acute MI; she is asymptomatic

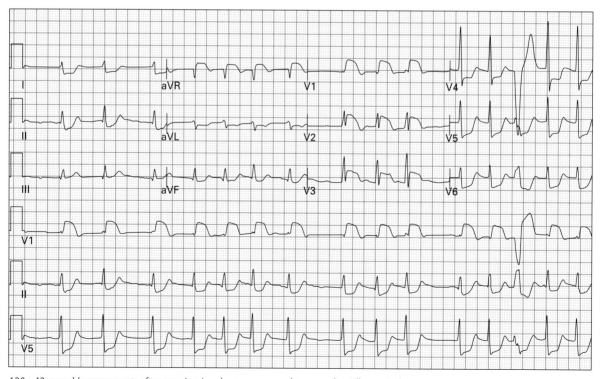

130. 42 year old man presents after experiencing chest pressure and syncope; he still reports chest pressure

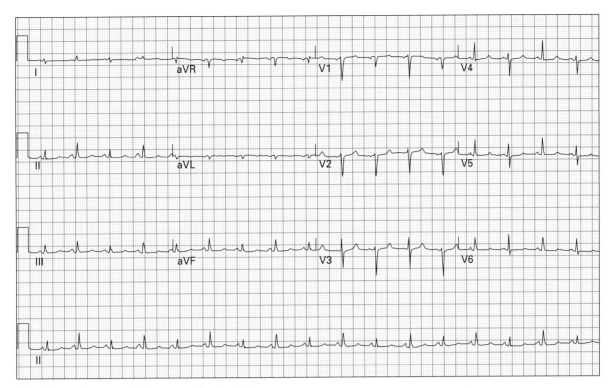

131. 50 year old woman with dyspnea and hypotension

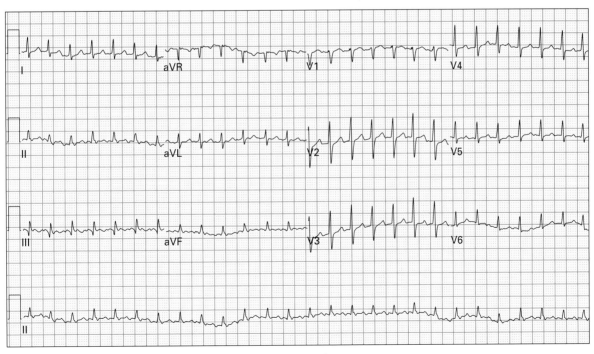

132. 55 year old man with dyspnea and palpitations one week after cardiac bypass surgery

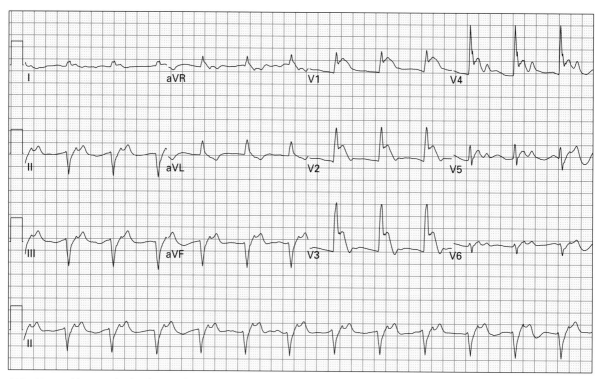

133. 81 year old man with a brief seizure followed by dyspnea and diaphoresis

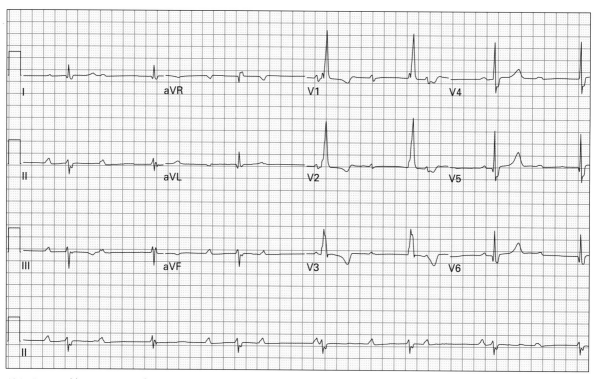

134. 51 year old man presents after a syncopal episode

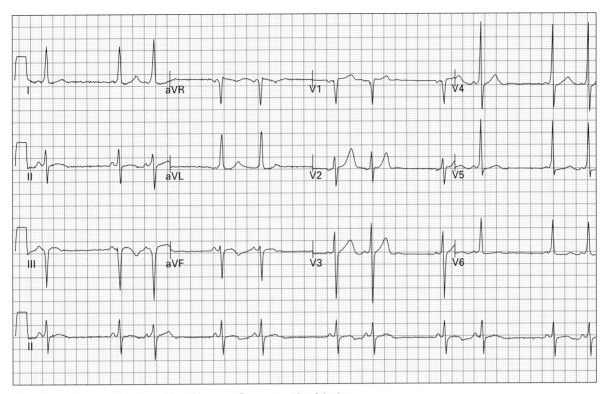

135. 39 year old man with history of "rapid heart rate" presents with palpitations

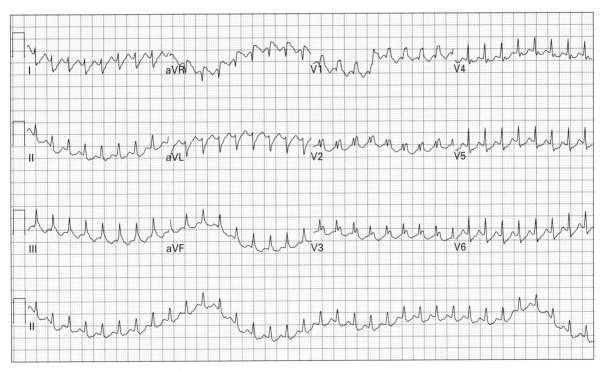

136. 46 year old woman with severe lightheadedness

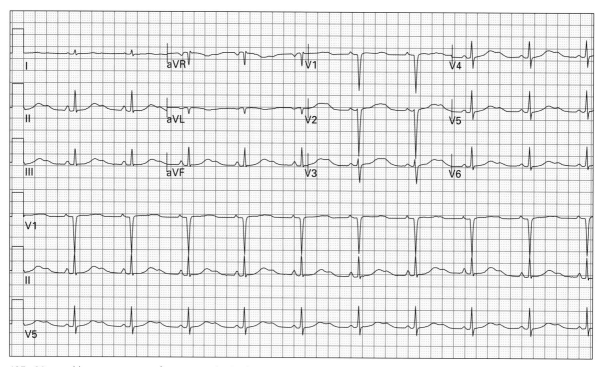

137. 39 year old woman presents after a syncopal episode

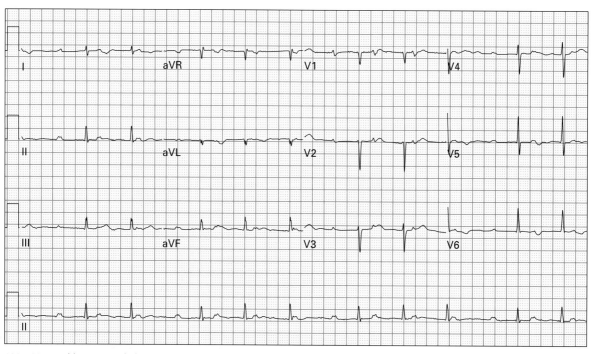

138. 66 year old woman with dyspnea and lightheadedness

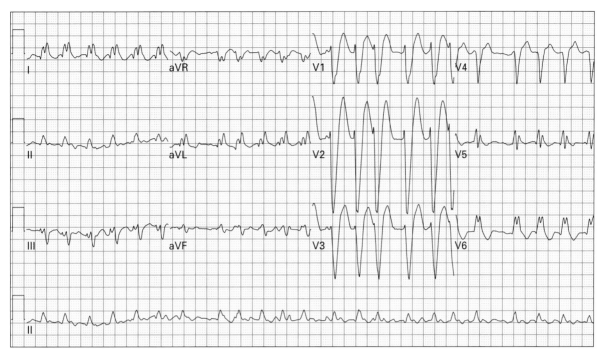

139. 60 year old man with diaphoresis and palpitations

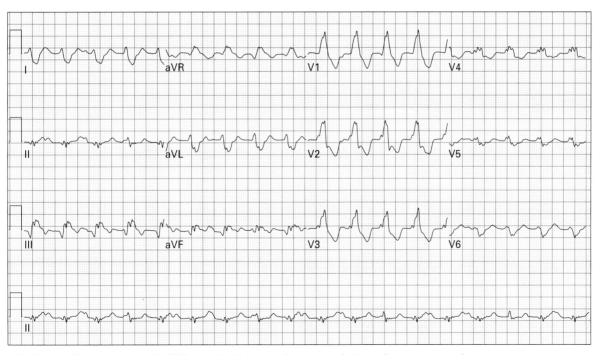

140. 58 year old man presents with mild dyspnea; he had severe chest pressure lasting an hour prior to arrival

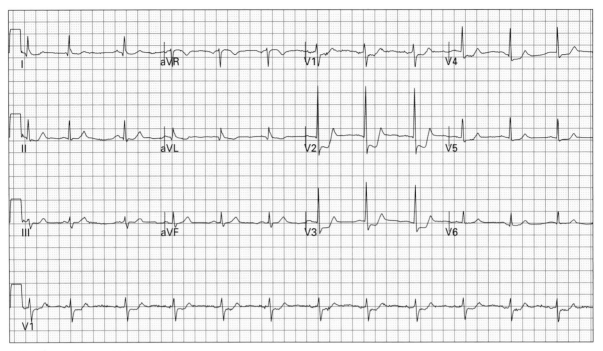

141. 66 year old man with chest and left arm pressure

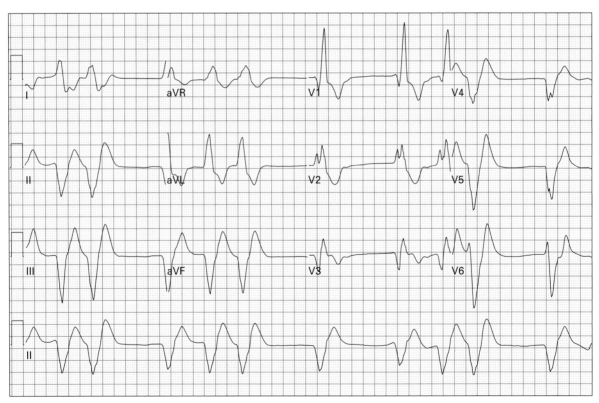

142. 65 year old woman with history of renal insufficiency presents lethargic with flu symptoms

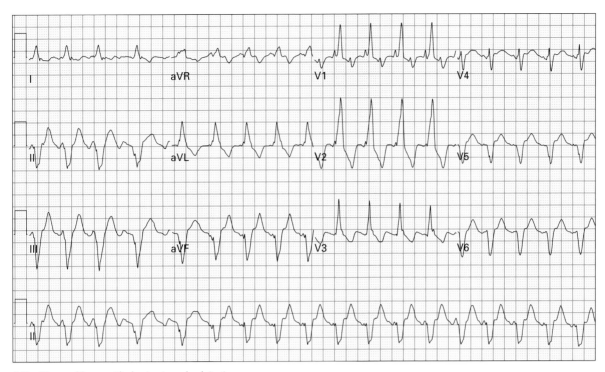

143. 63 year old man with chest pain and palpitations

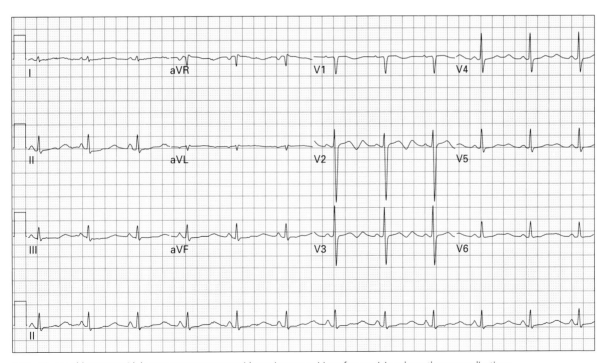

144. 46 year old woman with breast cancer presents with persistent vomiting after receiving chemotherapy medications

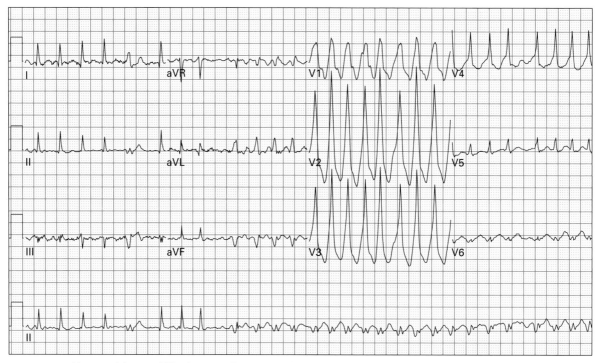

145. 61 year old man with history of "fast heart rates" presents with palpitations

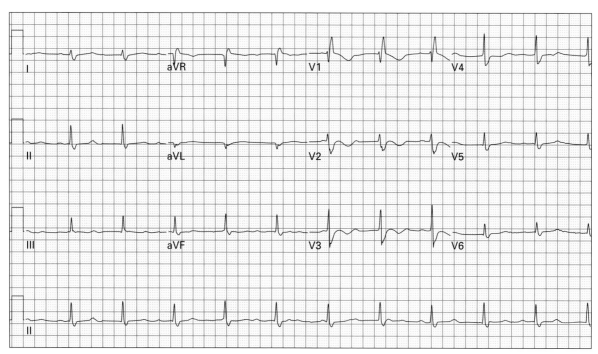

146. 29 year old man with HIV-related cardiomyopathy presents with generalized weakness

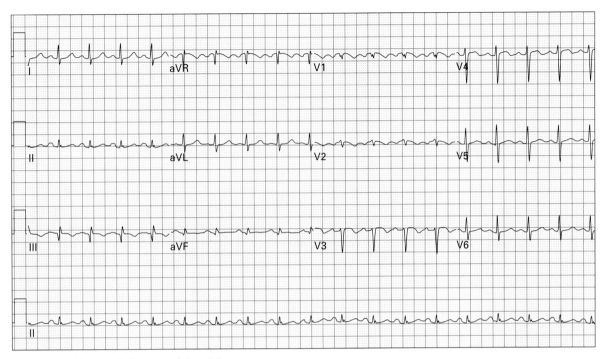

147. 53 year old man with dyspnea and chest tightness

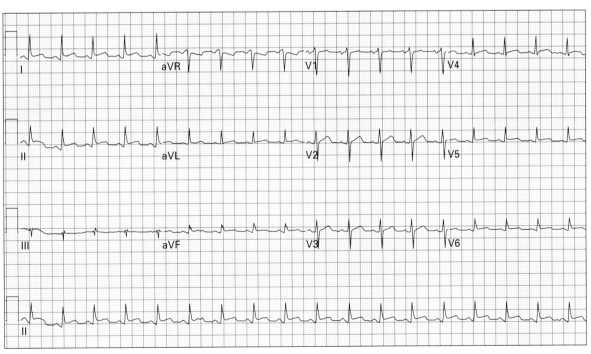

148. 42 year old man with pleuritic chest pain

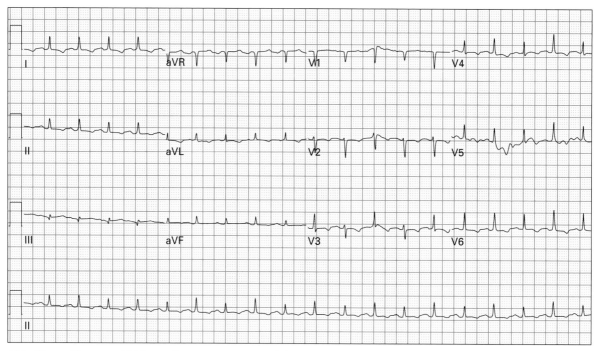

149. 48 year old woman with history of lung cancer presents with dyspnea and hypotension

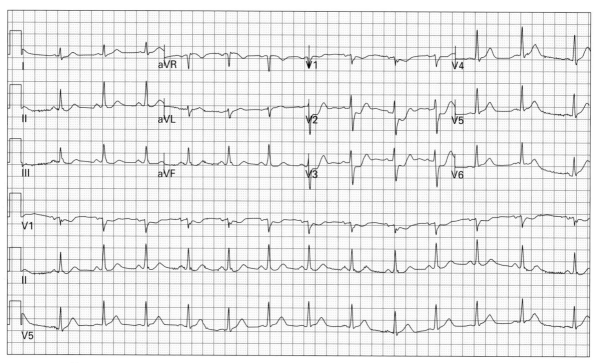

150. 58 year old man with chest pain, nausea, and diaphoresis

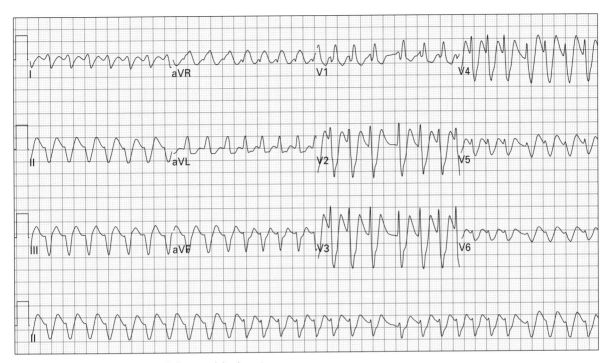

151. 67 year old man with lightheadedness and diaphoresis

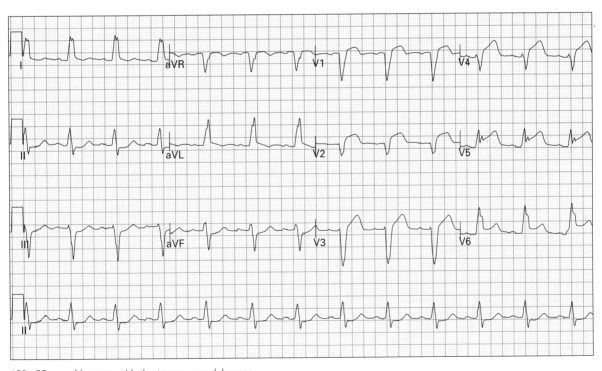

152. 57 year old woman with chest pressure and dyspnea

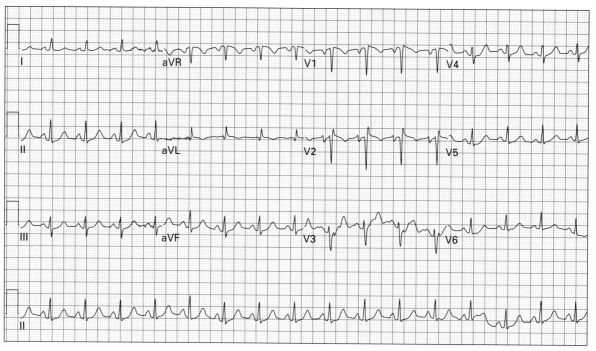

153. 38 year old woman presents after a syncopal episode

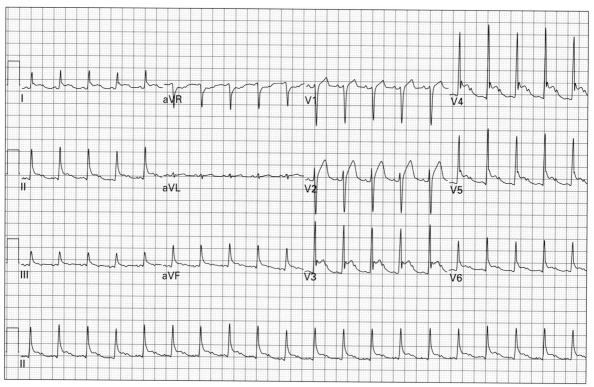

154. 43 year old man with sharp chest pain

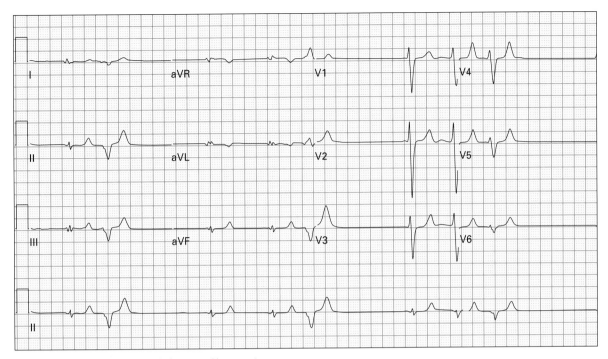

155. 38 year old woman presents lethargic and hypotensive

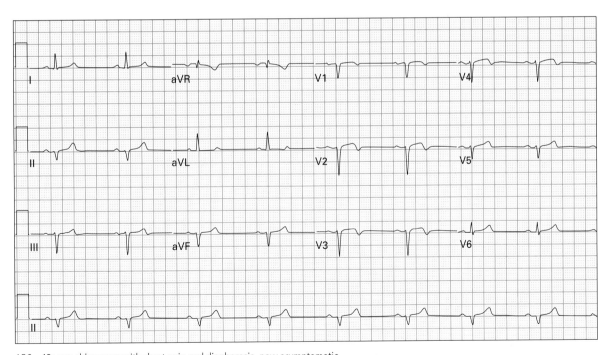

156. 43 year old woman with chest pain and diaphoresis, now asymptomatic

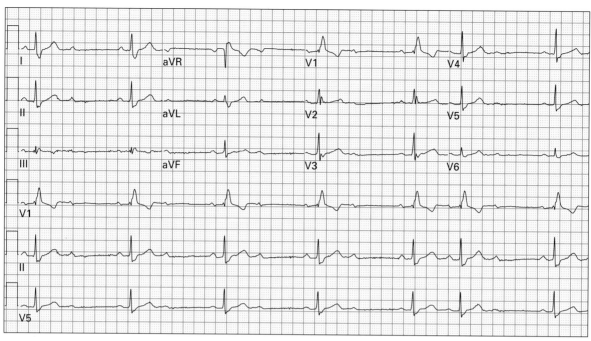

157. 88 year old man with dyspnea and severe lightheadedness

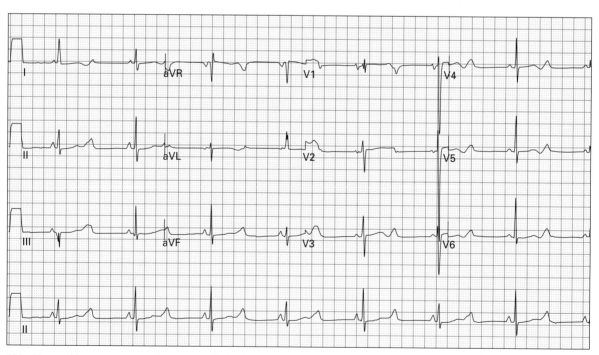

158. 58 year old woman presents after a syncopal episode

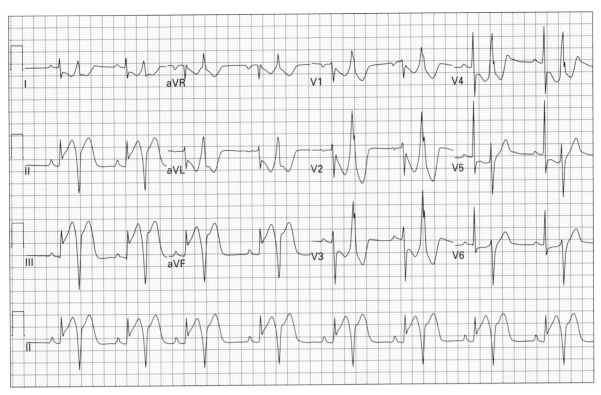

159. 47 year old woman with chest pressure and diaphoresis

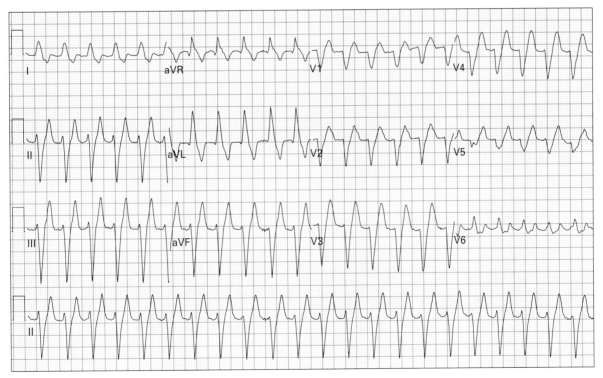

160. 72 year old man with fever and cough

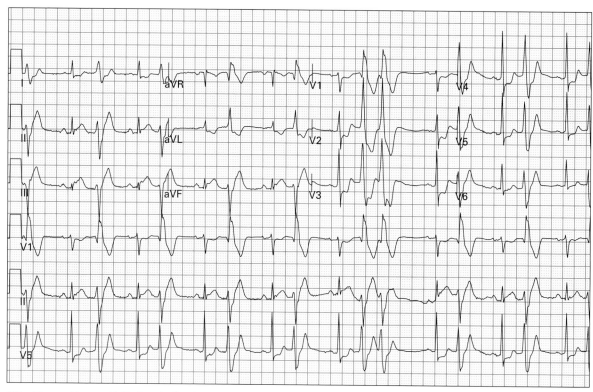

161. 50 year old man with "indigestion" and nausea

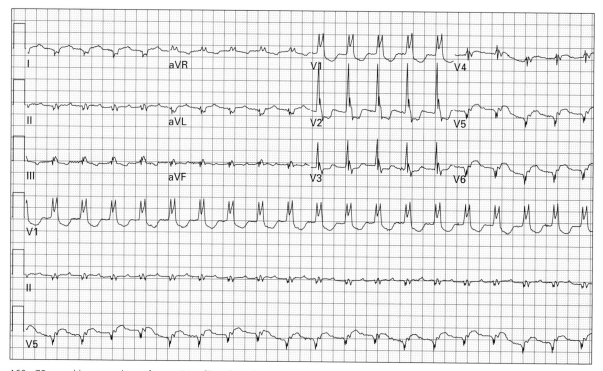

162. 78 year old man one hour after receiving fibrinolytics for acute MI

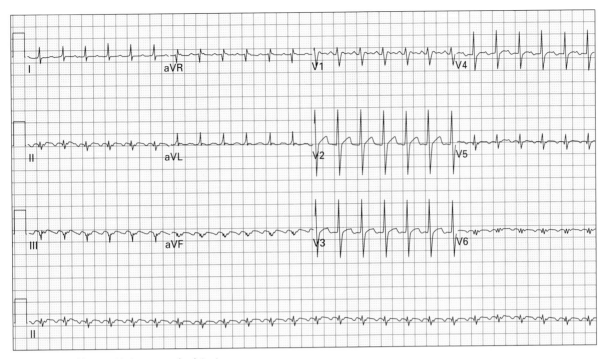

163. 68 year old man with dyspnea and palpitations

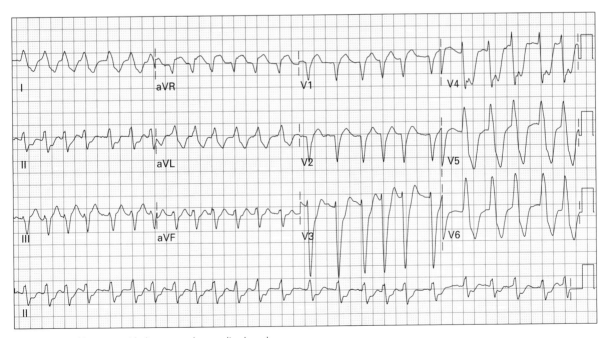

164. 90 year old woman with dyspnea and generalized weakness

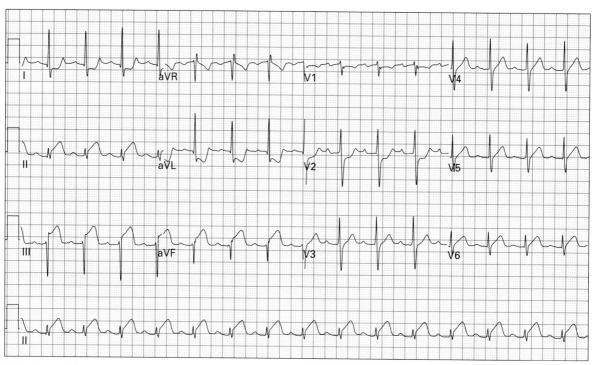

165. 71 year old man presents after syncopal episode, now with mild chest ache

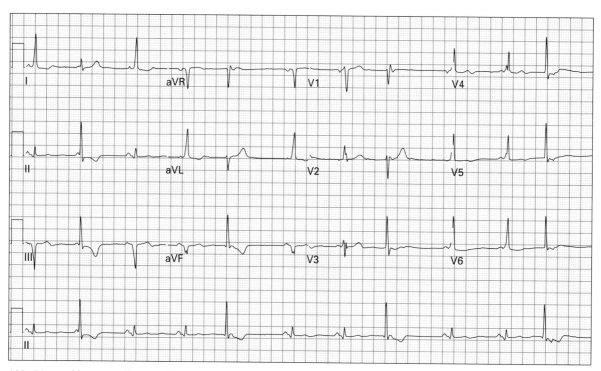

166. 76 year old woman with palpitations

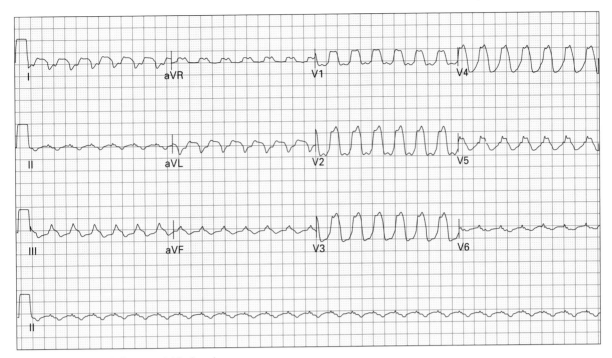

167. 55 year old man lethargic and dehydrated

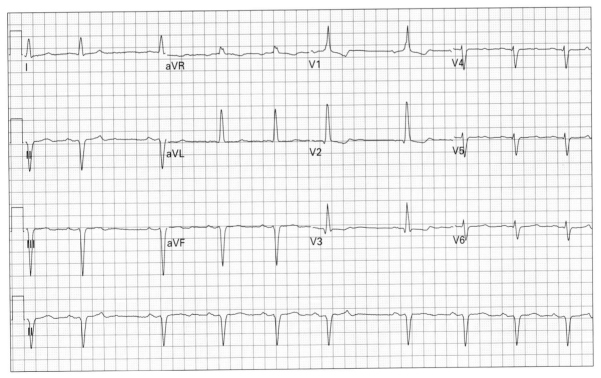

168. 92 year old woman with vomiting and diarrhea

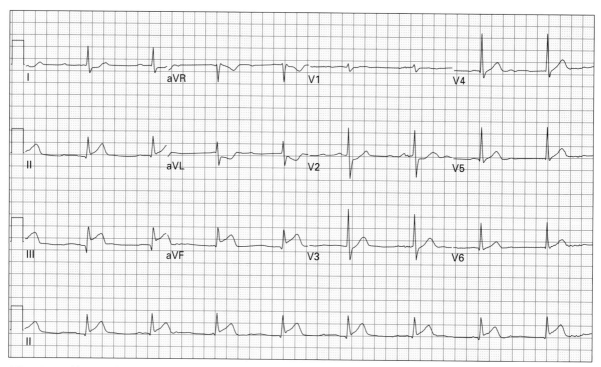

169. 49 year old man with chest pain and hypotension

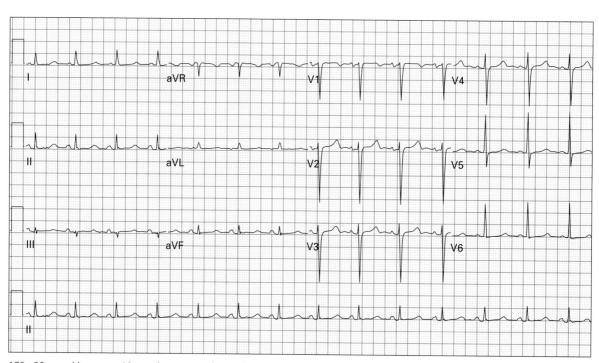

170. 39 year old woman with muscle cramps and paresthesias

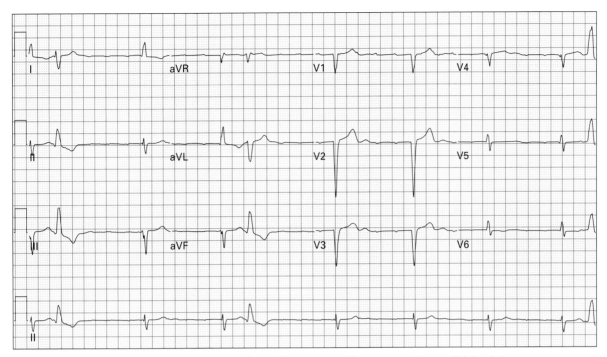

171. 93 year old man with history of chronic congestive heart failure presents with nausea, vomiting, and lightheadedness

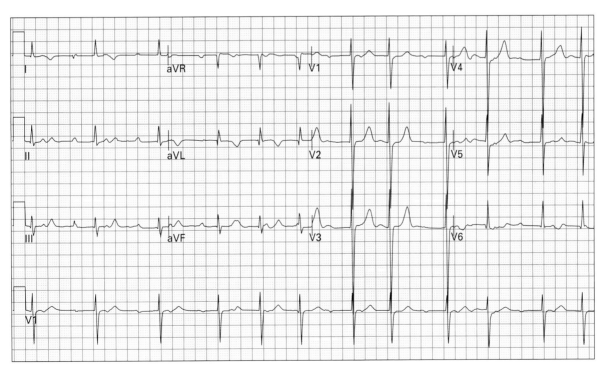

172. 49 year old man with chest tightness and lightheadedness

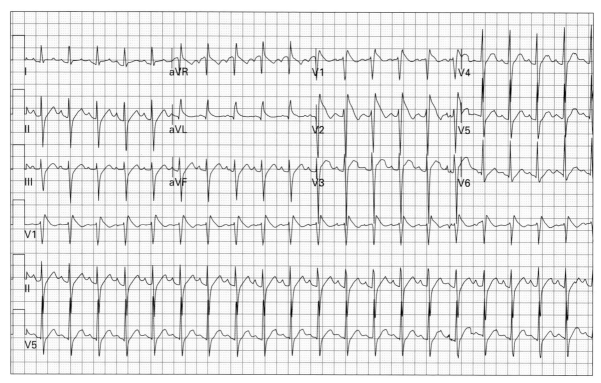

173. 20 year old man presents after witnessed cardiac arrest; pulse returned after one minute of chest compressions

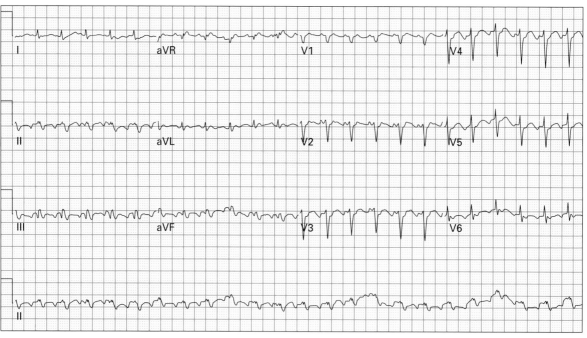

174. 83 year old woman with chest tightness and dyspnea

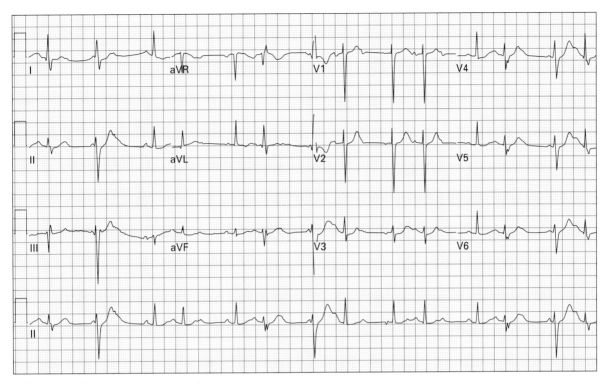

175. 76 year old woman with weakness and nausea

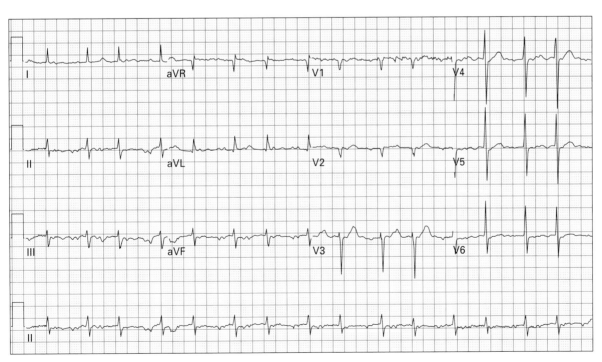

176. 64 year old man with lightheadedness

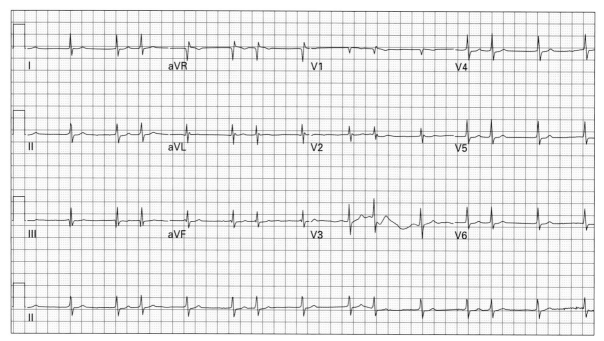

177. 56 year old woman with palpitations after taking a friend's blood pressure medication

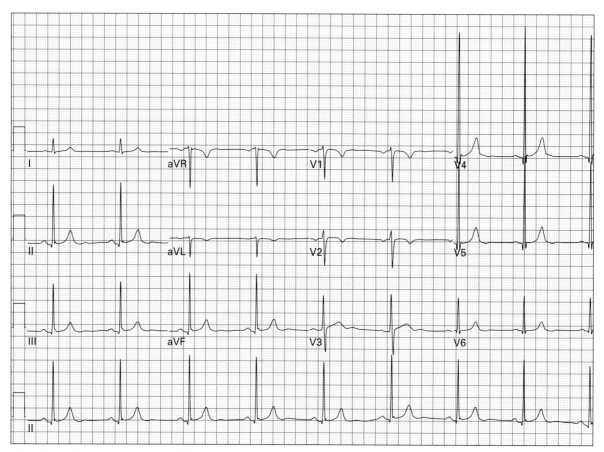

178. 58 year old with chest pressure and diaphoresis

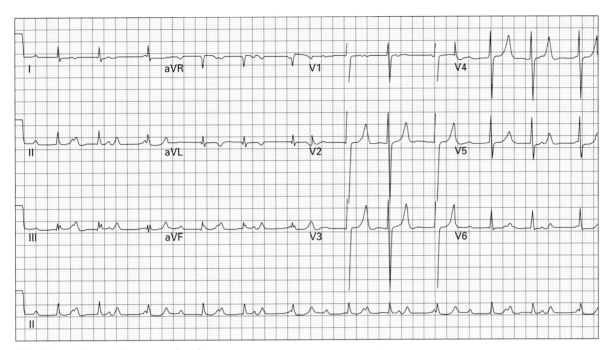

179. 48 year old man with nausea and weakness

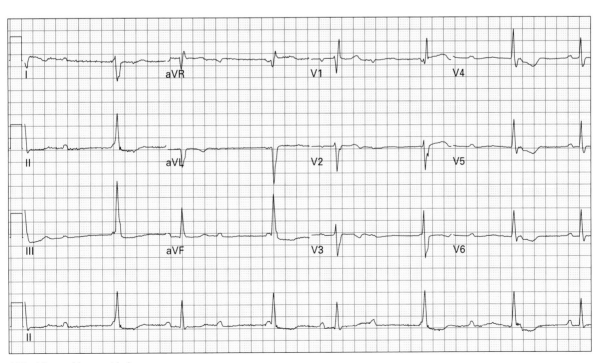

180. 46 year old man with dyspnea

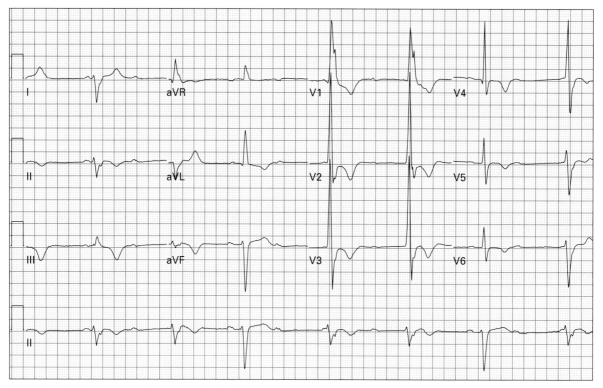

181. 71 year old man presents after a syncopal episode

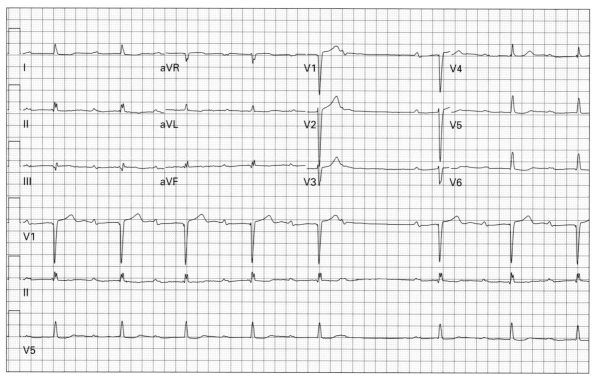

182. 74 year old man with a severe cardiomyopathy presents with exertional dyspnea; he recently began a new blood pressure medication

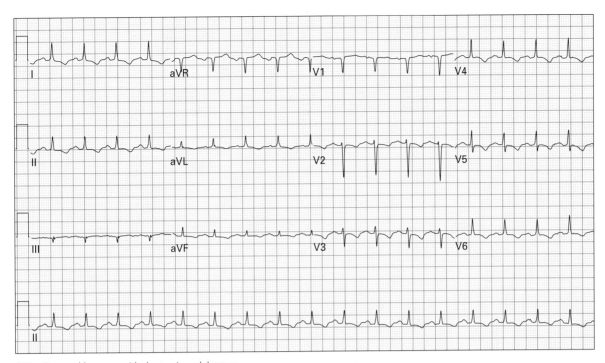

183. 49 year old woman with chest pain and dyspnea

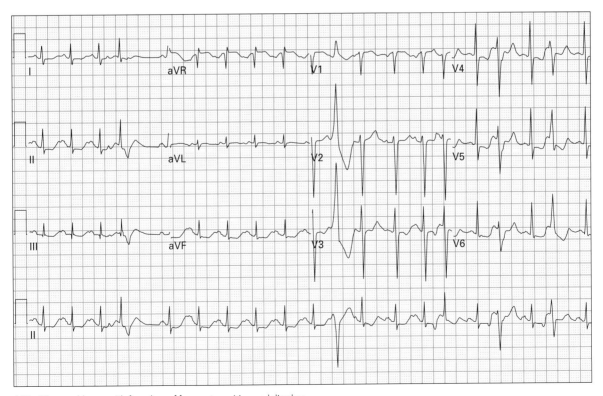

184. 62 year old man with four days of frequent vomiting and diarrhea

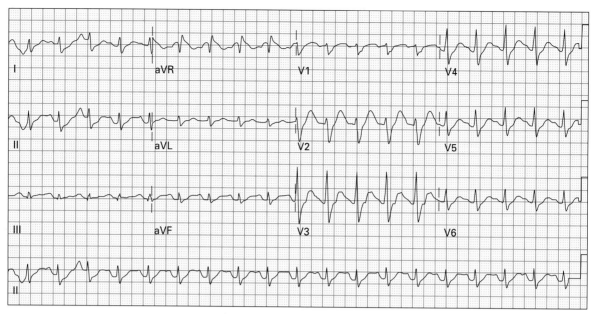

185. 41 year old man presents disoriented and incoherent

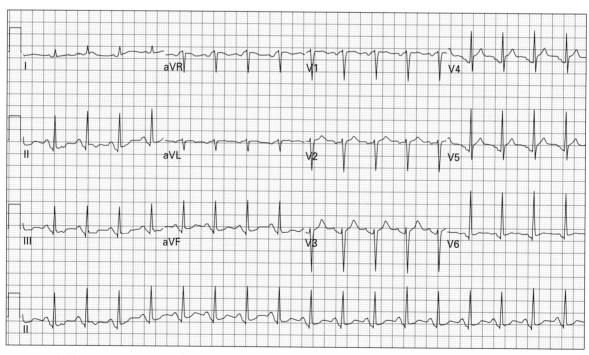

186. 53 year old woman with sharp chest pain and dyspnea

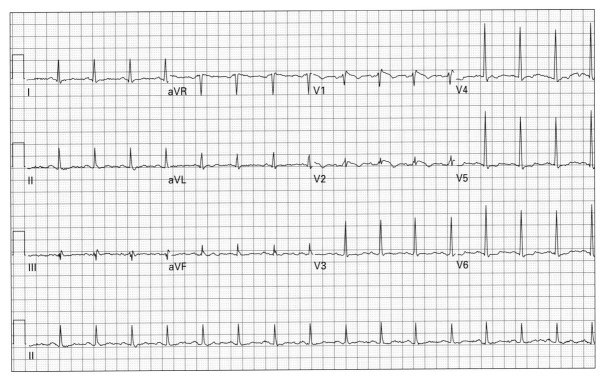

187. 46 year old man with two episodes of severe lightheadedness; now asymptomatic

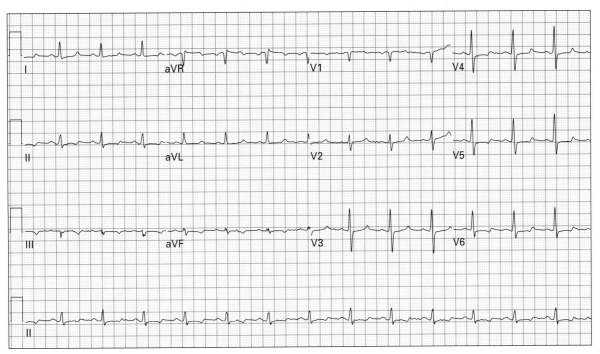

188. 44 year old man presents after a seizure

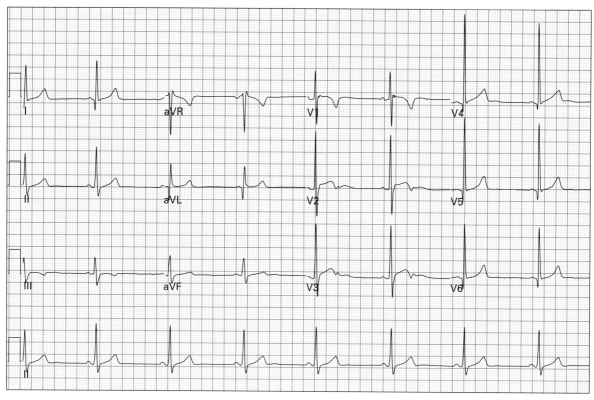

189. 29 year old man presents after a syncopal episode; now asymptomatic

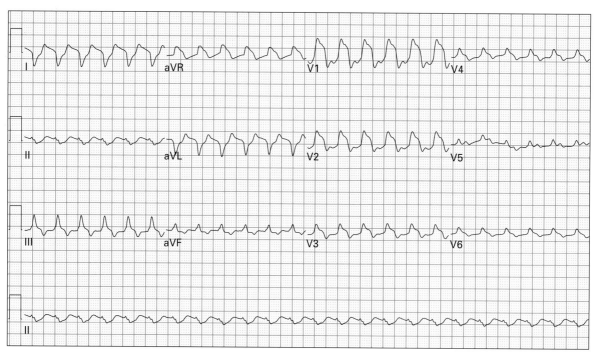

190. 55 year old woman presents with vomiting and lethargy

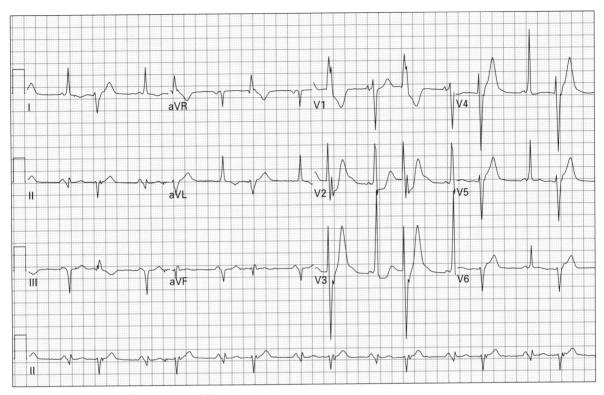

191. 77 year old woman with chest pain and dyspnea

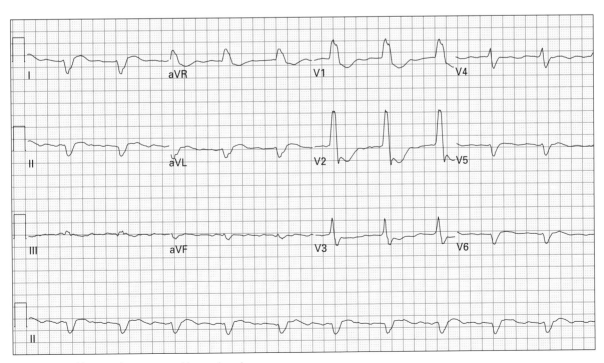

192. 54 year old man with nausea, vomiting, and weakness

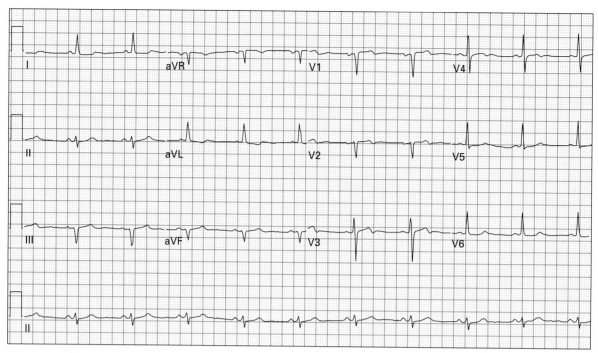

193. 53 year old man had "burning" chest pain and diaphoresis, now asymptomatic

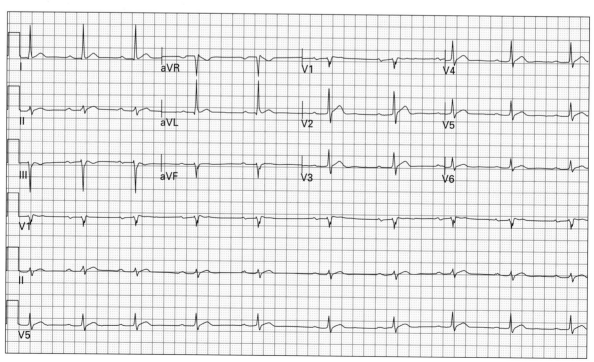

194. 69 year old man with nausea, vomiting, polyuria, and lethargy; he has a history of cancer

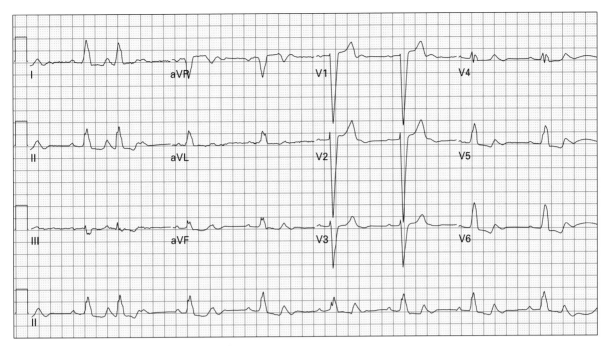

195. 65 year old woman presents with lightheadedness

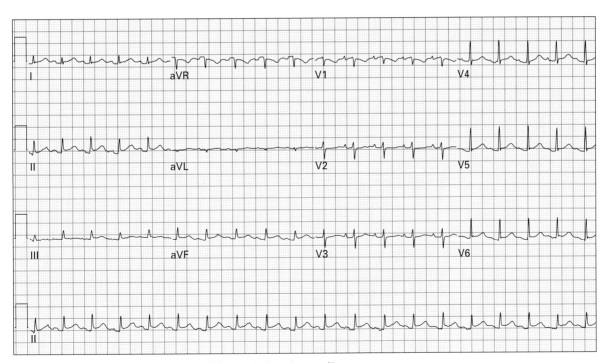

196. 55 year old man with chest heaviness and dyspnea; he has a history of lung cancer

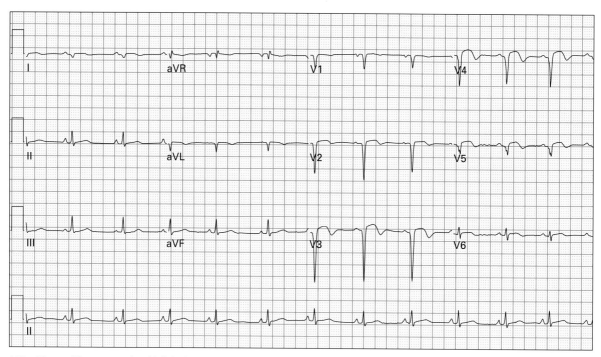

197. 46 year old man tripped and fell, hit head and now feels lightheaded; history of prior MI

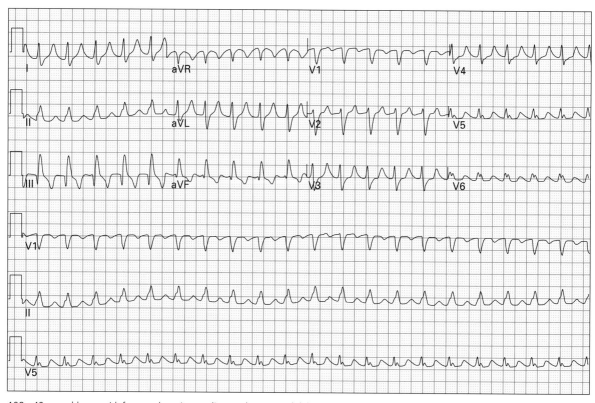

198. 42 year old man with fever and respiratory distress due to a multilobar pneumonia

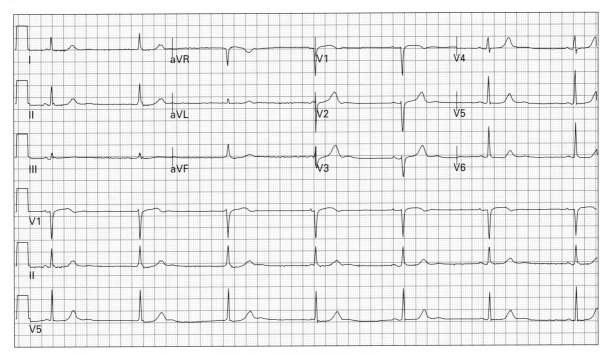

199. 54 year old woman presents after a syncopal episode; patient is still lightheaded

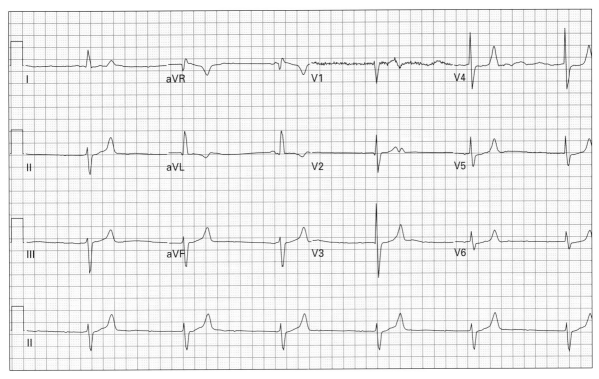

200. 50 year old man lethargic and hypotensive

ECG interpretations and comments

(Rates refer to ventricular rate unless otherwise indicated)

111. **SR with first degree AV block, rate 95, LBBB, ST-segment abnormality consistent with acute ischemia or MI.** LBBB is associated with characteristic repolarization abnormalities that all emergency physicians should know well. In all leads, ST-segments are displaced in an opposite direction to the terminal deflection of the QRS complex. The magnitude of this "discordance" is allowed to be up to 5 mm. Case #63 demonstrates LBBB with normal or expected discordance. In 1996, Sgarbossa[1] published a set of criteria which utilize this expected ST-segment discordance to make predictions about the chances of a patient with LBBB having an AMI. She stated that acute MI should be strongly considered in the presence of LBBB when any of the following apply: (1) ST-segment elevation ≥1 mm is concordant (in the same direction) with the QRS complex; (2) ST-segment depression of ≥1 mm is present in leads V1, V2, or V3 (i.e. concordant ST-segment depression in these leads); or (3) ST-segment elevation of ≥5 mm is discordant with the QRS complex. Although the sensitivity of any of these findings is low, the specificity (likelihood of ruling in for AMI) is extremely high, and the presence of any of these "Sgarbossa criteria" is now considered reasonable justification to provide immediate fibrinolytics or PCI to patients with LBBB and anginal symptoms (the presence of a *new* LBBB is also sufficient criteria to initiate these measures). This patient meets the Sgarbossa criteria in leads V2–V4, in which there is ≥5 mm of ST-segment elevation discordant with the QRS complex ("excessive discordance"). This patient did, in fact, rule in for acute MI based on positive cardiac biomarkers and a critical stenosis in the LAD artery. See figure below.

This figure corresponds to case #111. LBBB with evolving acute MI

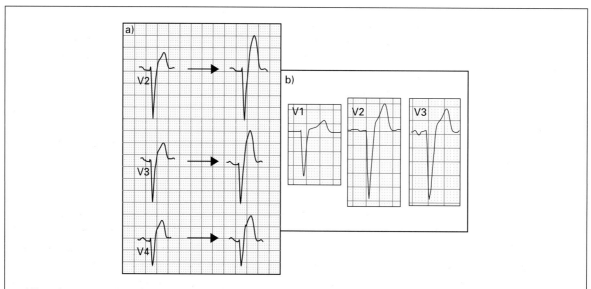

a) Note the progression of electrocardiographic abnormalities seen in this patient with acute MI and LBBB (20 minute interval). The degree of discordant STE is acceptable in the initial complexes; over the 20 minute time period, however, the degree of ST segment elevation greatly increases—in the appropriate clinical setting, this change suggests acute MI. b) Note the "normal" amount of discordant STE seen in these uncomplicated LBBB complexes.

112.   **SR with first degree AV block, rate 93, LBBB, ST-segment abnormality consistent with acute ischemia or MI.** Criteria for diagnosis of acute MI in the presence of LBBB were reviewed in the prior case. In this case, concordant STE ≥1 mm is present in lateral leads I, aVL, V5, and V6 consistent with acute MI. Excessive discordant STE >5 mm is also present in leads V1–V4.

This figure corresponds to case #112. LBBB with acute lateral MI

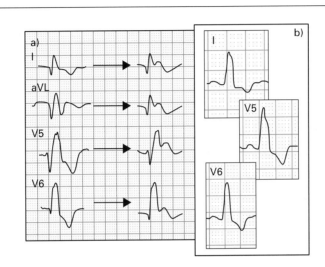

a) Progression of a lateral wall AMI in this patient with LBBB. Note the development of concordant STE in the lateral leads. b) Appropriate, or "normal," ST/T complexes in the lateral leads with the LBBB pattern. Note that the ST-segments and T-waves are discordant with respect to the QRS complex.

113.   **SR, rate 83, acute anterior-septal MI versus ventricular aneurysm.** The distinction between acute MI versus ventricular aneurysm is difficult. Both entities are associated with localized Q-waves and ST-segment elevation. Two additional ECG findings that very highly specific for acute MI include reciprocal ST-segment changes and prominent T-waves (often referred to as "hyperacute" T-waves). The absence of these findings certainly doesn't rule out acute MI but should at least warrant consideration of ventricular aneurysm as an alternative diagnosis. In this case, artifact obscures many of the ST-segments, however, the T-waves are "blunted" in size. The ECG is not diagnostic but at least suggestive of ventricular aneurysm. Acquisition of serial ECGs can also be helpful in clarifying matters, as acute MI is likely to demonstrate some evolving ST-segment or T-wave changes. Alternatively, bedside echocardiography is diagnostic. In this case, the echocardiogram confirmed a ventricular aneurysm. See figure on p. 166.

114.   **VT versus sodium channel blocker toxicity, rate 118.** At first glance, this wide QRS complex tachycardia without obvious P-waves would appear to be VT. However, on closer inspection, the rhythm is slightly irregular, with rates <120/minute in some areas. VT is a very regular rhythm (unless fusion or capture beats are present, although they demonstrate varying morphology), and rarely presents with a rate <120/minute. "Mimics" of VT should therefore be considered. A common mimic of VT is accelerated idioventricular rhythm, but this is most commonly found as a reperfusion rhythm following treatment of acute MI. The other common mimics of VT are toxic and metabolic (e.g. hyperkalemia), both of which commonly present at lower rates than VT and they may also demonstrate slight irregularity. Although some of the leads (e.g. lead aVR) have a near sine-wave appearance, other leads demonstrate QRS complexes that have a more "normal" appearance and, in these leads, prominent

This figure corresponds to case #113. Left ventricular aneurysm

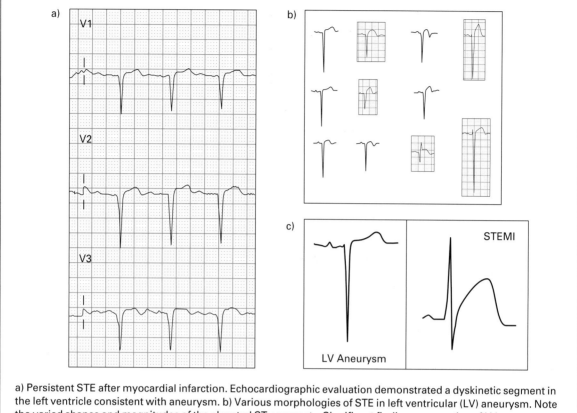

a) Persistent STE after myocardial infarction. Echocardiographic evaluation demonstrated a dyskinetic segment in the left ventricle consistent with aneurysm. b) Various morphologies of STE in left ventricular (LV) aneurysm. Note the varied shapes and magnitudes of the elevated ST-segments. Significant findings suggestive of LV aneurysm are Q-waves and T-waves of diminished height. c) A comparison of LV aneurysm and the STE of acute MI. Note the diminished T-wave height relative to the QRS complex in LV aneurysms. In the LV aneurysm, the QRS complex is markedly larger than the T wave; with acute MI, the T-wave assumes a larger relative size compared to the QRS complex.

T-waves that would be expected with hyperkalemia are absent. This patient did respond to treatment with intravenous sodium bicarbonate and it was later discovered that she had overdosed on medications with sodium-channel blocking effects.

115. **ST, rate 146, acute anterior-lateral MI.** The rhythm strip (figure a)) and 12-lead ECG demonstrate QRS complexes that appear wide and regular, giving the impression of VT. However, P-waves are present with every QRS complex, consistent with ST. Furthermore, some leads (e.g. leads II, aVF, V2) clearly demonstrate narrow QRS complexes and reveal the fact that it is actually profound ST-segment deviation that is mimicking wide QRS complexes. Massive STE such as that seen in this case is easily misdiagnosed as VT when the entire 12-lead ECG is not scrutinized. STE is found in the anterolateral leads and reciprocal ST-segment depression is found in the inferior leads. See figure opposite.

116. **Atrial flutter with variable AV conduction, ventricular rate 185, left posterior fascicular block (LPFB).** Atrial flutter with rapid ventricular conduction is the most frequently misdiagnosed tachydysrhythmia. Flutter waves are often inverted in the inferior leads and are therefore easily overlooked or discounted as artifact; it seems that our eyes are more trained to detect upright atrial waves than inverted ones. Therefore, before ruling out atrial

This figure corresponds to case #115

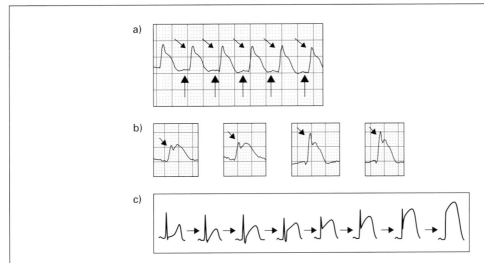

a) The rhythm strip demonstrates an apparent wide QRS complex tachycardia at a rate of 146/minute. A rapid review of this rhythm strip could suggest ventricular tachycardia in an ill-appearing patient. Actually, this is a narrow complex tachycardia in a patient with an acute MI. The large arrows indicate the P-waves and the small arrows the R-waves of the QRS complexes. b) The apparent wide QRS complexes result from giant R-waves fusing with massively elevated ST-segments. This structure is formed when, in leads with prominent R-waves, the ST-segments elevate rapidly, obliterating the distinction of the QRS complex from the ST-segment—forming essentially a giant R-wave. Note here four examples of the giant R-wave with the arrow indicating the R-wave. c) The transition from a normal ST-segment to giant R-ST complex in a patient with rapidly evolving acute MI. Note the progressive rise in the ST-segment with greater obliteration of the QRS complex–ST-segment differentiation, ultimately producing an apparent wide QRS complex.

flutter in patients with tachydysrhythmias, the authors recommend a simple maneuver to increase the yield in detecting flutter waves: turn the ECG upside down and re-examine the inferior leads. The figure below demonstrates this point—when the ECG is inverted, the flutter waves in lead aVF appear more prominent visually because they are now "upright." The two other causes of an irregular narrow QRS complex tachydysrhythmia (atrial fibrillation and MAT) are therefore excluded. A rightward axis is noted, for which the differential diagnosis includes LPFB, lateral MI, right ventricular hypertrophy, acute or chronic lung disease (e.g. pulmonary embolism or emphysema, respectively), ventricular ectopy, hyperkalemia, sodium-channel blocker drug toxicity, and misplaced leads. LPFB is diagnosed based on the presence of a rightward axis, rS complexes in leads I and aVL, and qR complexes in lead III.

This figure corresponds to case #116. "Flutter waves" in this atrial flutter with variable conduction

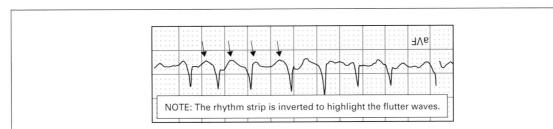

NOTE: The rhythm strip is inverted to highlight the flutter waves.

Note that the flutter waves (arrows) are more easily seen in lead aVF when the tracing is inverted.

117. **MAT, rate 145, occasional aberrantly conducted complexes, acute inferior-anterior-lateral MI, non-specific IVCD.** The rhythm is irregularly irregular with P-waves of at least three morphologies, indicating MAT. Some QRS complexes have a slightly different morphology, likely the result of mild aberrant conduction. STE is present in the anterior, lateral, and (to a lesser extent) inferior leads indicating ongoing injury. Q-waves indicative of infarction have already developed in the inferior and lateral leads. Leftward axis is attributable to inferior MI. Non-specific IVCD is diagnosed based on slight widening of the QRS complex (100 msec).

118. **SR, rate 90, occasional PVCs, LBBB, ST-segment abnormality consistent with acute ischemia or MI.** LBBB is associated with characteristic repolarization abnormalities that all emergency physicians should know well. In all leads, ST-segments are displaced in an opposite direction to the terminal deflection of the QRS complex. Case #63 demonstrates LBBB with normal or expected discordance. Sgarbossa[1] has published a set of criteria which utilize this expected ST-segment discordance to make predictions about the chances of a patient with LBBB having an AMI. These criteria are described in detail in case #111. This patient meets the Sgarbossa criteria in lead V2, in which there is ≥5 mm of ST-segment elevation discordant with the QRS complex ("excessive discordance"). Additionally, although the ST-segment depression in the inferior leads does not meet the Sgarbossa criteria, those leads should also be a cause for concern. In each of inferior leads, the terminal deflection of the QRS complex is downwards, and the ST-segments are concordant (depressed). Note that even in lead II, in which the major portion of the QRS complex is upwards, the *terminal* deflection is downwards. This patient had positive cardiac biomarkers, and he was found to have a 100% LAD artery occlusion as well as significant stenosis in the right coronary artery.

119. **Atrial tachycardia with second degree AV block type 1 (Wenckebach, Mobitz I) and 3:2 conduction, ventricular rate 115, incomplete RBBB.** This rhythm was initially misdiagnosed at atrial fibrillation because of its irregularity. However, close inspection reveals that the rhythm is actually *regularly* irregular. Regular irregularity of the cardiac rhythm, whether in the setting of a bradycardia or tachycardia, should prompt consideration of a second degree AV block. Lead V1 reveals distinct atrial activity at a rate of 172. A 3:2 atrial:ventricular contraction ratio occurs; prolongation of the PR-interval is noted from the first P-QRS complex to the next, then the third atrial contraction is non-conducted and followed by a pause before the cycle repeats. Although second degree AV block usually occurs in conjunction with bradydysrhythmias, Mobitz I also occasionally occurs in the presence of tachydysrhythmias, a fact that is not well known. As a result, these rhythms are often misdiagnosed as rapid atrial fibrillation. Recognizing that these rhythms are *regularly* irregular provides a major clue to the proper diagnosis.

120. **Atrial fibrillation, ventricular rate 190, WPW.** Atrial fibrillation is diagnosed based on the profound irregularity of the rhythm. The classic delta waves of WPW are not reliably present when the rhythm is anything other than SR. However, the presence of WPW with atrial fibrillation here is unmistakeable for two reasons: (1) The QRS complexes vary in width and morphology. This occurs because some of the atrial impulses are conducted through the normal His-Purkinje system producing narrow QRS complexes, some are conducted through the accessory pathway producing wide QRS complexes, and some QRS complexes are a fusion between both type of conduction. (2) Although the overall rate is approximately 190 beats/minute, some areas of the ECG demonstrate a rate approaching 250–300 beats/minute. The accessory pathway is capable of conducting at exceedingly rapid rates. In contrast, atrial fibrillation in the absence of an accessory pathway doesn't usually demonstrate such variability in the QRS morphology, and the rate rarely exceeds 180 beats/minute. The distinction between normal atrial fibrillation versus atrial fibrillation with WPW is critical. Normal atrial fibrillation is usually treated with AV-nodal blocking medications (e.g. calcium channel blockers, beta-adrenergic blockers, amiodarone, digoxin, etc.). However, the use of AV-nodal blocking medications in atrial fibrillation with WPW facilitates conduction through the accessory pathway, resulting in a paradoxical acceleration of the ventricular and rapid cardiovascular collapse.

This figure corresponds to case #120. Atrial fibrillation in the Wolff-Parkinson-White syndrome

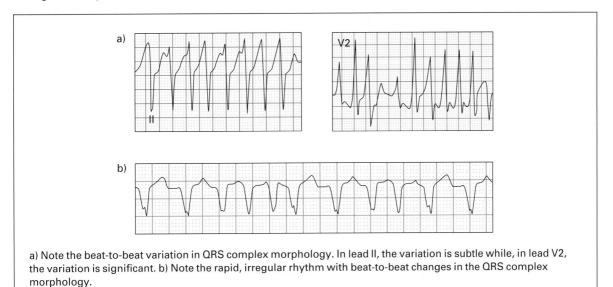

a) Note the beat-to-beat variation in QRS complex morphology. In lead II, the variation is subtle while, in lead V2, the variation is significant. b) Note the rapid, irregular rhythm with beat-to-beat changes in the QRS complex morphology.

Procainamide is considered safe in this setting, although perhaps the safest and most reliable acute treatment for rapid atrial fibrillation with WPW is electrical cardioversion. This patient was hemodynamically stable, probably because he was young and otherwise healthy. He was treated with intravenous procainamide, after which he was admitted for ablation of the accessory pathway. See figure above.

121. **SR with second degree AV block type 1 (Wenckebach, Mobitz I), rate 47, persistent juvenile T-wave pattern.** Mobitz I may sometimes be found in healthy young patients with high vagal tone, especially athletes, as was the case with this patient. In the absence of concerning symptoms or signs, this AV block doesn't require treatment. T-wave inversions are noted in leads V1–V3. Children and adolescents have a slight posterior orientation of the T-waves, which often results in T-wave inversions in these leads. By adulthood, the T-wave orientation becomes more anterior producing upright T-waves in V2–V3 (the T-waves in lead V1 often remain inverted or flat). However, young adults, especially women, may have a persistence of the "juvenile T-wave pattern." Diagnosis of this normal variant should only be made if the T-wave inversions are asymmetric and shallow. If the inversions are symmetric in shape, ≥3 mm deep, or occur in patients >45–50 years of age, anteroseptal myocardial ischemia should be assumed.

122. **Probable SR with first degree AV block, rate 97, IVCD likely due to hyperkalemia.** The rhythm is regular. SR is presumed, though cannot be definitely diagnosed in the absence of upright P-waves in leads I, II, III, and aVF. P-waves are best found in leads V1–V2 with a pronounced first degree AV block. The QRS complexes have a markedly wide, bizarre morphology. A rightward axis is present with wide S-wave in the lateral leads and a prominent R-wave complex in lead V1, producing an RBBB-type of appearance. The T-waves are also prominent. All of these findings are typical of severe hyperkalemia. Hyperkalemia is well-known to produce myriad of ECG abnormalities, including new fascicular blocks or bundle branch blocks and axis changes. A new rightward axis is especially common in cases of severe hyperkalemia. This patient's serum potassium level was 9.2 mEq/L (normal 3.5–5.3 mEq/L). The patient's mental status was likely caused by a marked metabolic acidosis, which commonly accompanies severe hyperkalemia. See figure on p. 170.

This figure corresponds to case #122. Markedly widened QRS complexes, diminished P waves, and prolonged PR-intervals in a patient with profound hyperkalemia

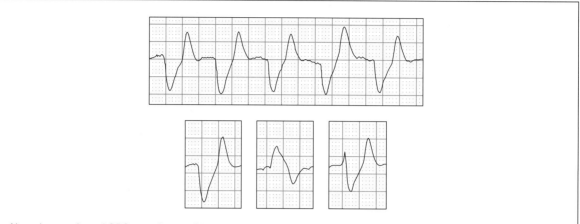

Note the very broad QRS complexes with a duration of 200 msec. This QRS complex is approaching that encountered in the sinoventricular rhythm of profound hyperkalemia.

123. **SR, rate 70, U-waves suggestive of hypokalemia, prolonged QT-interval.** Prominent U-waves are present in the precordial leads producing a "camel hump"[2] effect with the T-wave. This T-U fusion complex (see figure opposite), which tends to be most prominent in the mid-precordial leads, is highly suggestive of moderate-to-severe hypokalemia. In contrast, the inferior leads more often demonstrate T-wave flattening and the appearance of a prolonged QT-interval in the setting of moderate-to-severe hypokalemia. Although hypokalemia is often listed as a cause of a prolonged QT-interval, the appearance of prolongation is actually caused by the U-wave. As a result, some authors do not include hypokalemia in the differential diagnosis of QT-interval prolongation. This patient's serum potassium level was 1.6 mEq/L (normal 3.5–5.3 mEq/L).

124. **SR, rate 88, intermittent episodes of non-sustained VT, T-wave abnormality consistent with inferior and anteroseptal ischemia, consider pulmonary embolism.** The underlying sinus rate is 88, but episodic non-sustained VT (defined as VT lasting less than 30 seconds and not associated with hemodynamic compromise) at a rate of 175 beats/minute interrupts the SR. Retrograde P-waves are noted just after the ventricular complexes. Other abnormalities that are easily overlooked in the setting of the unusual rhythm are the rightward axis (large S-wave in the intrinsic first complex of lead I) and the T-wave inversions in the right precordial leads as well as in inferior leads III and aVF. This combination of findings, especially the T-wave inversions, is far more specific for acute pulmonary embolism than cardiac ischemia.[3] This patient was found to have a massive pulmonary embolism. The ventricular dysrhythmia resolved without specific antidysrhythmic therapy.

125. **SR with first degree AV block, rate 90, bifascicular block (RBBB + LPFB), inferior and anterolateral ischemia, consider sodium-channel blocking drug toxicity or overdose.** A rightward axis is present. The differential diagnosis for rightward axis includes LPFB, lateral MI (due to large Q-waves), RVH, acute (e.g., pulmonary embolism) and chronic (e.g., emphysema) lung disease, ventricular ectopy, hyperkalemia, overdoses of sodium-channel blocking drugs (e.g., cyclic antidepressants), and misplaced leads. Normal or slender adults with a horizontally posititioned heart can also demonstrate a rightward QRS axis. This patient meets criteria for LPFB (rS in leads I and aVL, qR in III). The usual cause of a LPFB is coronary artery disease. In this 15 year old girl with no presumed prior heart disease, however, one must consider alternative causes of a new LPFB pattern: hyperkalemia

This figure corresponds to case #123. The U-wave of hypokalemia

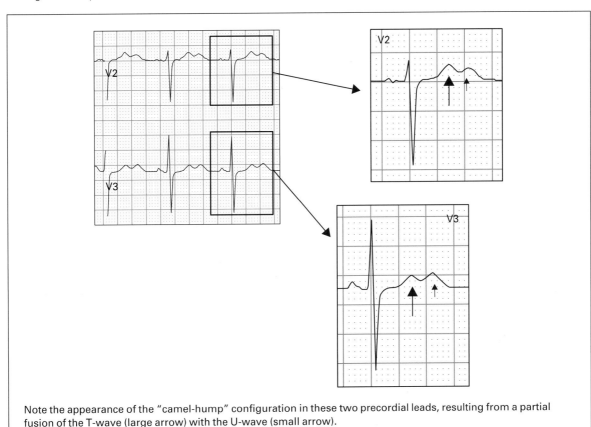

Note the appearance of the "camel-hump" configuration in these two precordial leads, resulting from a partial fusion of the T-wave (large arrow) with the U-wave (small arrow).

and sodium-channel blocking drug toxicity. Both conditions are well-known to induce a new rightward axis and fascicular block pattern. Hyperkalemia can probably be excluded based on the absence of prominent T-waves. History later revealed that the patient had tried to commit suicide by ingesting multiple tricyclic antidepressant medication pills. The patient was treated with sodium bicarbonate which resulted in resolution of the bifascicular block as well as the ST-segment depression.

126. **SR, rate 80, incomplete RBBB with STE in septal leads suggestive of the Brugada syndrome.** The Brugada syndrome was first described by Brugada[4] in 1992. Patients with the Brugada syndrome, despite structurally normal hearts, tend to develop sudden monomorphic or (more often) polymorphic VT (causing sudden death if persistent, syncope if self-terminating). The *exact* cause is not certain, but it appears to be related to sodium channel dysfunction. Definitive diagnostic study and treatment (placement of an internal cardioverter-defibrillator) is done in the electrophysiology laboratory, but there are ECG abnormalities which are highly suggestive that all emergency physicians should know. The ECG typically demonstrates an incomplete or complete RBBB pattern in leads V1–V2 with STE. The morphology of the STE may be convex upwards or straight (as in this case), or concave upwards. The convex or straight morphology is more sensitive and specific for the diagnosis. The ECG of Brugada syndrome can be distinguished from that of an acute AMI with RBBB because reciprocal ST-segment depression is generally absent in patients with Brugada syndrome. Clinical information is helpful in the distinction as well—patients with Brugada syndrome usually present after having symptoms suggestive of an aborted tachydysrhythmia (e.g. syncopal episode, palpitations, etc.) rather than anginal symptoms. See figure on p. 172.

This figure corresponds to case #126. Brugada syndrome

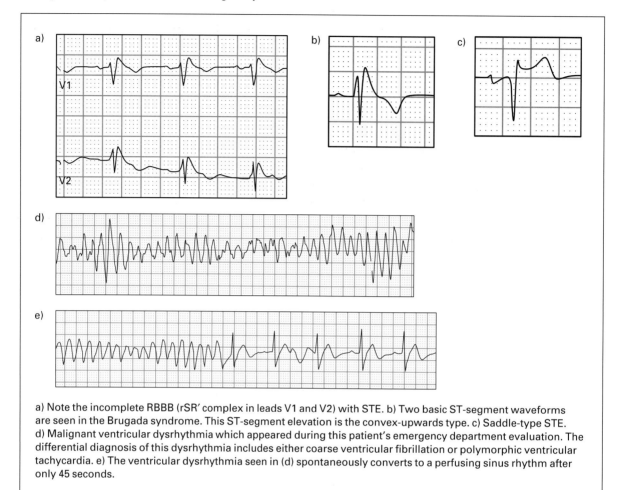

a) Note the incomplete RBBB (rSR' complex in leads V1 and V2) with STE. b) Two basic ST-segment waveforms are seen in the Brugada syndrome. This ST-segment elevation is the convex-upwards type. c) Saddle-type STE. d) Malignant ventricular dysrhythmia which appeared during this patient's emergency department evaluation. The differential diagnosis of this dysrhythmia includes either coarse ventricular fibrillation or polymorphic ventricular tachycardia. e) The ventricular dysrhythmia seen in (d) spontaneously converts to a perfusing sinus rhythm after only 45 seconds.

127. **Atrial fibrillation/flutter, ventricular rate 150, occasional aberrantly conducted complexes versus fusion complexes, bifascicular block (RBBB + LAFB), anterolateral ischemia.** The rhythm is mostly irregular, consistent with atrial fibrillation. However, small areas of the rhythm are regular (e.g. the final five beats). This likely represents sections of atrial flutter. Atrial fibrillation and atrial flutter commonly co-exist like this. The terminal portion of the QRS complexes in some leads, such as lead V3, give the appearance of retrograde P-waves. However, it is actually part of the QRS complex, a fact that becomes obvious when the QRS complexes above in lead V2 are compared for duration. The 1st, 6th, and 16th QRS complexes have a slightly different morphology. This is likely the result of either increased aberrancy in those complexes or possibly the result of a fusion between an intrinsic beat and a PVC. Despite the slight variation in QRS morphology, this ECG should not be confused with that of atrial fibrillation with WPW (see case #120). Atrial fibrillation with WPW is associated with far more variation of the QRS morphology and is also associated with rates approaching 250–300 beats/minute in some areas. On the current ECG, the rate never gets that fast.

128. **SB, rate 55, HLVV, non-specific T-wave abnormality in inferior leads, abnormal Q-waves in lateral leads suggestive of hypertropic cardiomyopathy (HCM).** HCM is a common cause of sudden death in adolescents

and young adults. The characteristic ECG findings include: (1) large-amplitude QRS complexes (HLVV), especially in the precordial leads; (2) tall R-waves in the right precordial leads that mimic posterior MI or RVH; and (3) deep narrow Q-waves in the inferior (occasional) or lateral (more common) leads. HLVV is the most sensitive finding, and the abnormal Q-waves are the most specific. These Q-waves are often mistakenly diagnosed as MI of undetermined age. However, these are *not* infarction-type Q-waves. The Q-waves associated with MI should be at least 40 seconds in duration. The Q-waves of HCM are very deep and *narrow*. Non-specific T-wave abnormalities are common with HCM and are present in the inferior leads here. HCM was confirmed in this patient during Doppler echocardiography, the definitive diagnostic modality.

129. **Accelerated idioventricular rhythm (AIVR), rate 90.** Ventricular escape rhythms, also known as "idioventricular rhythms," are usually associated with rates 20–40 beats/minute. When a ventricular rhythm is 40–120 beats/minute, it is referred to as an *accelerated* idioventricular rhythm. The diagnosis of VT is reserved for ventricular rhythms ≥120 beats/minute. This patient's rhythm strip demonstrates P-waves unassociated with the QRS complexes, AV dissociation, typical of ventricular rhythms (see figure below). AIVR is commonly found in the setting of AMI, especially after the administration of fibrinolytic agents. AIVR is thought to be a marker of reperfusion. Antidysrhythmic therapy is unnecessary, and may in fact induce asystole. AIVR in itself is not a hemodynamically destabilizing rhythm, and usually is self-terminating within minutes, as was the case here.

This figure corresponds to case #129. Accelerated idioventricular rhythm

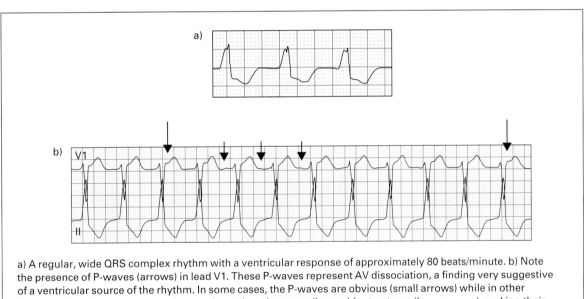

a) A regular, wide QRS complex rhythm with a ventricular response of approximately 80 beats/minute. b) Note the presence of P-waves (arrows) in lead V1. These P-waves represent AV dissociation, a finding very suggestive of a ventricular source of the rhythm. In some cases, the P-waves are obvious (small arrows) while in other instances, the P waves are superimposed on other electrocardiographic structures (large arrows), making their identification more difficult. Note that these P-waves are not seen in lead II.

130. **Atrial fibrillation, ventricular rate 90, occasional PVCs, acute anterior-septal MI.** Pronounced STE is present in leads V1–V3, consistent with acute MI. The J-point is so elevated, in fact, that it gives an appearance of an incomplete RBBB with convex upward STE like that found in Brugada syndrome. The presence of reciprocal ST-segment depression in the inferior and lateral leads, however, leaves no doubt that this patient is suffering from a large acute MI.

131. **ST, rate 105, low voltage and electrical alternans suggestive of pericardial effusion.** This ECG has all three of the classic findings of large pericardial effusion: (1) low QRS voltage, (2) tachycardia, and (3) electrical alternans. Although electrical alternans is often considered the most characteristic, in reality it is present in fewer than one-third of cases of large pericardial effusions and pericardial tamponade. On the other hand, the combination of low voltage and tachycardia is more common. When the low voltage is known to be a new finding compared to prior ECGs, the combination is very specific for large pericardial effusions. The only other entity that reliably causes *new* low voltage would be a large *pleural* effusion, a diagnosis that can easily be confirmed or excluded on routine chest radiography. Although there are various published ECG criteria for the diagnosis of low voltage, a simple definition of low voltage is when the amplitudes of the QRS complexes in all of the limb leads is <5 mm or when the amplitudes of the QRS complexes in all of the precordial leads is <10 mm. The differential diagnosis for low voltage includes large pericardial effusions, large pleural effusions, myxedema, end-stage cardiomyopathy, severe chronic obstructive pulmonary disease, obesity, infiltrative myocardial diseases (e.g. sarcoid, amyloid), constrictive pericarditis, and prior massive MI. This patient was found to have a large pericardial effusion with tamponade due to a pericardial metastasis.

This figure corresponds to case #131. Pericardial effusion

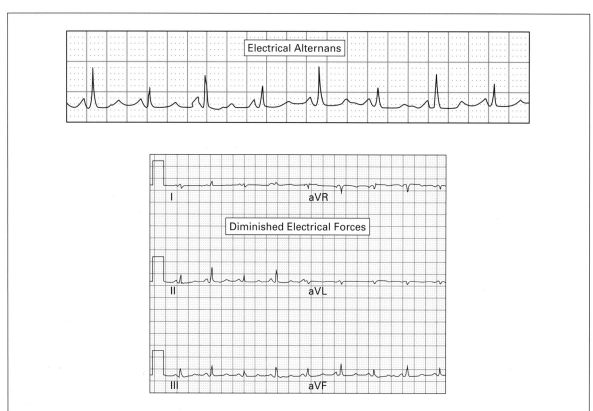

The electrocardiographic triad for pericardial effusion includes electrical alternans, diminished electrical forces (low QRS voltage), and tachycardia.

132. **Atrial flutter with 2:1 AV conduction, ventricular rate 160.** Atrial flutter with rapid ventricular conduction is the most frequently misdiagnosed tachydysrhythmia. When the ventricular response is rapid, flutter waves are commonly obscured by the QRS complexes or T-waves resulting in misdiagnosis as ST, atrial fibrillation, or SVT.

Complicating matters further, flutter waves are often inverted in the inferior leads and are therefore easily over-looked or discounted as artifact; it seems that our eyes are more trained to detect upright atrial waves than inverted ones. Therefore, as described in case #116, the authors recommend a simple maneuver to increase the yield in detecting flutter waves: turn the ECG upside down and re-examine the inferior leads. When the ECG is inverted, flutter waves in lead II at a rate of 320 beats/minute suddenly appear more prominent to the eyes. This patient was initially misdiagnosed as having ST, and he was treated for several hours with intravenous fluids in the hopes of reducing his heart rate. When there still was no change in the heart rate, the ECG was more closely scrutinized and the proper diagnosis was made. This patient also has somewhat low voltage in the limb leads, although not meeting formal criteria as described in case #131. He was found to have a moderate-sized pericardial effusion, a complication of his recent surgery.

133. **Accelerated AV junctional rhythm, rate 76, acute inferior-anterior-septal MI, incomplete RBBB, LAFB.** When normal P-waves are absent in a regular rhythm, distinction must be made between an AV junctional rhythm versus a ventricular rhythm. In this particular case, the significant ST-segment abnormality gives the appearance of a wide-QRS complex rhythm, which might suggest a ventricular origin. However, examination of the lateral leads gives the best measure of the true QRS complex duration, clearly <120 msec. Therefore an AV junctional rhythm is probable. The intrinsic rate of an AV junctional pacemaker is 40–60 beats/minute. This rhythm is faster, therefore it is termed an *accelerated* AV junctional rhythm. Retrograde P-waves are noted immediately following the QRS complexes, especially in the inferior leads. STE is present in the inferior and anteroseptal leads consistent with acute MI. The tall R-wave in lead V1 is presumed to be caused by an incomplete RBBB, and criteria for LAFB (leftward axis, qR in I and aVL, rS in III) is present as well. This patient's incomplete RBBB and LAFB were old, but the ST-segment changes and rhythm were new. His seizure was attributed to cerebral hypoperfusion due to acute MI.

134. **SR with AV dissociation and third degree heart block, junctional escape rhythm, rate 40, bifascicular block (RBBB + LAFB).** The sinus rate is 62 beats/minute and regular, and the ventricular rate is 40 beats/minute and regular. The atrium and ventricle are functioning independent of each other indicating AV dissociation. There is no evidence that any of the P-waves are being conducted to the ventricle, thus third degree ("complete") heart block is diagnosed. The escape rhythm of 40 beats/minute is typical of either a junctional or ventricular rhythm, The QRS complexes are wide. Wide QRS complexes can be caused by ventricular beats, aberrant intraventricular conduction (e.g. bundle branch block), WPW, electronic pacemakers, hyperkalemia, hypothermia, and an assortment of medications. In this case, the wide QRS complexes have a typical RBBB morphology (rsR' in V1, wide S-waves in I, V5, and V6). A LAFB is present as well. T-wave inversions and slight ST-segment depression in the right precordial leads are common in the presence of a RBBB. Small q-waves in the lateral leads are present but are too narrow to be considered diagnostic of a previous lateral MI—infarction-related q-waves should be at least 40 msec in duration.

135. **SR with frequent PACs in a pattern of atrial bigeminy, rate 62, WPW.** Grouped beats are almost always caused by either second degree AV block (Mobitz I or II) or by the presence of PACs. PACs are often overlooked, but in fact they are the most common overall cause of pauses on an ECG rhythm—always look closely for a PAC just prior to the pause. The pause occurs as the sinus node must "reset." In this case, second degree AV block is easily ruled out by the lack of non-conducted P-waves. The second beat in each pair is the result of a PAC. The P-wave in the second beat has a *slightly* different morphology, best appreciated in leads V1 and V2. The patient has a short PR interval (<120 msec), slight prolongation of the QRS complex, and delta waves (slurred upstroke of the QRS complex) best noted in the lateral leads. This triad is classic for WPW. WPW is also responsible for the leftward axis. This patient had a history of episodes of a rapid heart rate, had been non-compliant with follow-up, and he did not know he had WPW.

136. **SVT, rate 200, incomplete RBBB, LPFB.** The three major considerations in patients with narrow QRS complex (<120 msec) tachycardias are SVT, atrial flutter, and sinus tachycardia. Neither flutter waves nor sinus P-waves are noted, excluding the latter two possibilities. Small retrograde P-waves are noted immediately following the QRS complexes in many of the leads, a finding that is common with certain types of SVTs. A RBBB QRS morphology is noted in the right precordial leads with wide S-waves in the lateral leads, but the QRS complex is <120 msec; therefore the diagnosis of an *incomplete* RBBB is made. LPFB is diagnosed based on a rightward axis, rS complexes in leads I and aVL, and qR complexes in lead III. ST-segment depression is present in the inferior and lateral leads, a common finding in patients with SVT. This ST-segment depression is often assumed to indicate ischemia, but it actually does not correlate with stress testing and its relevance is unknown.

137. **SR, rate 60, U-waves suggestive of hypokalemia, prolonged QT-interval.** The patient has a markedly prolonged QT-interval and a "camel hump"[2] appearance of the T-waves especially in the precordial leads. This is caused by the presence of U-waves fused to the terminal portion of the T-wave, a finding highly suggestive of moderate-to-severe hypokalemia. Whether hypokalemia truly is a cause of QT-interval prolongation or whether the appearance of the QT-prolongation should simply be attributed to the fusion of the T-wave and U-wave is perhaps just a matter of semantics. Patients with hypokalemia are at risk for dysrhythmias, not unlike patients with "true" QT-interval prolongation. This patient developed torsade de pointes soon after this ECG was performed (see rhythm strip in figure below). She was resuscitated successfully and found to have a serum potassium level of 2.0 mEq/L (normal 3.5–5.3 mEq/L). After potassium replacement, her U-waves resolved and she did well.

This figure corresponds to case #137

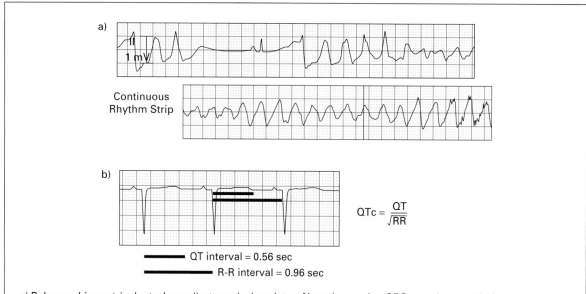

$$QTc = \frac{QT}{\sqrt{RR}}$$

QT interval = 0.56 sec

R-R interval = 0.96 sec

a) Polymorphic ventricular tachycardia, torsade de pointes. Note the varying QRS complex morphology and amplitude with polarities changing from positive to negative. b) With review of the 12-lead ECG, the diagnosis of torsade de pointes is diagnosed with demonstration of a prolonged QT-interval. The QT-interval can be assessed via two separate methods. The most simple method involves a comparison of the QT-interval to the R-R interval. If the QT-interval is longer than one-half of the R-R interval, then the QT-interval is too long for that particular heart rate. This method should be used when the patient is in sinus rhythm with rates ranging from 60 to 100/minute. The second method involves the Bazett formula. Here, the QTc-interval (corrected QT-interval) is calculated using the measured QT and R-R intervals. With values greater than 0.45 sec, a prolonged QT-interval is diagnosed.

138. **SR with second degree AV block type 1 (Wenckebach, Mobitz I), rate 66, PRWP, lateral ischemia.** The sinus rate is 88. In the rhythm strip, the first two P-waves are conducted with a markedly prolonged PR-interval. The third P-wave, occurring just after the second QRS complex, is the non-conducted P-wave. The cycle then resumes with a 4:3 AV conduction ratio. PRWP, defined as an R-wave in lead V3 <3 mm in height, indicates a possible prior anteroseptal MI. Inverted T-waves in the lateral leads suggest lateral wall ischemia.

139. **Atrial fibrillation/flutter, ventricular rate 138, non-specific IVCD.** The rhythm overall is irregular suggesting atrial fibrillation, but co-existent atrial flutter accounts for the more regular rhythm at the beginning of the rhythm strip; flutter waves can also be seen in various areas of the rhythm strip as well. Atrial fibrillation and atrial flutter are well-known to co-exist and tend to be treated similarly. The QRS complexes are markedly wide. The broad S-waves in the right precordial leads have the appearance of a LBBB. However, formal diagnostic criteria for LBBB do not allow for the small q-waves in lateral leads I, V5, and V6. Rather, true LBBB is characterized by large monophasic R-waves in these leads. Therefore the diagnosis of non-specific IVCD is made instead. Rules of discordance and concordance have been described for acute MI in LBBB (see case #111), but they have not been clearly described for patients like this with an LBBB-like IVCD. The "excessive discordance" noted in lead V2 should be cause for concern, but this patient would *not* be a candidate for immediate fibrinolytics. All emergency physicians should be familiar with the Sgarbossa criteria[1] for diagnosis of acute MI in the presence of LBBB; but we must be equally familiar with diagnostic criteria that rule in *and rule out* LBBB before we apply Sgarbossa's crititeria.

140. **AIVR, rate 106.** This is a wide QRS complex regular rhythm without evidence of regular sinus activity. Two diagnostic possibilities exist in such a case: a junctional rhythm with aberrant conduction (given the morphology of lead V1, RBBB would be a consideration) versus a ventricular rhythm. The presence of AV dissociation, which is best seen in the lead II rhythm strip (see figure below), virtually confirms that this is a ventricular rhythm. A rightward axis is present, the differential diagnosis of which includes ventricular ectopy, LPFB, lateral MI, RVH, acute (e.g. pulmonary embolism) or chronic (e.g. emphysema) lung disease, hyperkalemia, sodium-channel blocking medication toxicity, and misplaced leads. In this case the rightward axis is further evidence in favor of a ventricular rhythm. Because the rate is faster than the normal intrinsic rate of ventricular pacemakers (i.e. 20–40 beats/minute), this rhythm is referred to as an accelerated ventricular rhythm, or "accelerated idioventricular rhythm." When the rate is >120 beats/minute, VT is diagnosed. AIVR is commonly a sign of reperfusion following acute MI, and probably occurred because this patient developed spontaneous reperfusion of an acute MI. His cardiac biomarkers were markedly positive and he had evidence of diffuse coronary occlusions on his cardiac catheterizations. AIVR in and of itself is not a dangerous rhythm—it does not induce hemodynamic instability, and it usually terminates spontaneously within minutes as it did in this case. The danger arises when the treating physician mistakenly diagnoses VT and administers ventricular antidysrhythmics, which are well-known to cause these patients to develop asystole.

This figure corresponds to case #140

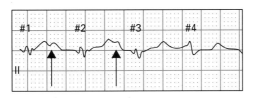

AV dissociation in this lead II rhythm strip confirms a ventricular source of this wide QRS complex tachycardia. With a rate of 106, an accelerated idioventricular rhythm is diagnosed. The P-waves (arrows) are seen following QRS complexes #1 and #2, providing evidence of AV dissociation; in complexes #3 and #4, the P-waves are obscured by the T wave.

141. **SR, rate 70, occasional PACs, acute posterior MI.** The majority of acute posterior MIs occur in the presence of a concurrent inferior wall or occasionally in the presence of a lateral wall MI. In those cases, the diagnosis of acute MI is easily made based on the "routine" findings in the inferior or lateral leads, and the treatment is essentially no different just because of the posterior extension of the MI. However, approximately 5% of posterior MIs occur in isolation, without STE in the inferior or lateral leads. These patients are candidates for immediate reperfusion therapy via PCI or fibrinolytics, even though there is no STE on the standard 12-lead ECG. Therefore, all emergency physicians should be comfortable with the diagnostic criteria for isolated acute posterior MI. In the right precordial leads (V1–V3), look for (1) horizontal ST-segment depression, often 2 mm or more; (2) large R-waves that increase in size over hours; and (3) upright T-waves. The use of posterior leads (see case #44) can confirm posterior infarction. The posterior leads in such cases will demonstrate findings typical of an STE MI: (1) STE, (2) Q-waves that increase in size over hours, and (3) inverted T-waves.

142. **Probable atrial fibrillation, ventricular rate 65, LVH, RBBB, possible metabolic abnormality or drug toxicity, prominent T-waves suggestive of hyperkalemia.** An exact interpretation of this unusual ECG is difficult. Atrial fibrillation is suspected given the irregularity. LVH is diagnosed based on R-wave amplitude in aVL >11 mm. RBBB is diagnosed based on the rsR' pattern in the right precordial leads and wide S-waves in lead I, V5, and V6. The most prominent abnormality is the width of the QRS complexes. QRS-interval prolongation to 200 msec or more is strongly suggestive of a metabolic abnormality (especially severe acidosis or severe hyperkalemia) or severe drug toxicity (especially drugs with sodium-channel blocking effects). The most common emergency department cause of bizarre, wide QRS complex rhythms is severe hyperkalemia. This patient was found to have a serum potassium level of 9.0 mEq/L (normal 3.5–5.3 mEq/L). Hyperkalemia is capable of producing a multitude of ECG abnormalities: unusual bradydysrhythmias, AV blocks, or tachydysrhythmias, ST-segment changes, axis changes, fascicular blocks, bundle branch blocks, and T-wave abnormalities. As a general rule, the more bizarre the ECG appears, the more strongly one should consider hyperkalemia.

143. **Atrial tachycardia with 2:1 AV conduction, ventricular rate 115, occasional fusion complexes, inferior and lateral MI of undetermined age, RBBB.** This ECG was initially interpreted as ST because several leads, especially lead V4, appear to show a 1:1 P:QRS ratio. However, on further inspection, atrial beats at a rate of 230/minute can be found in lead V1. Because the lead V1 electrode is positioned almost directly over the sinus node, this lead often provides the best evidence for sinus node activity and often demonstrates P-waves when no other leads do. The atrial activity here is termed "tachycardia" rather than "flutter" because the rate is <250 beats/minute. Leftward axis is present and is attributed to the presence of a prior inferior wall MI. Atrial beats fused to the initial portion of the QRS complex in the inferior leads give a false appearance of small r-waves in some complexes. The fourth QRS complex has a slightly different morphology and is probably a fusion of a conducted beat with a PVC.

144. **SR, rate 69, U-waves suggestive of hypokalemia, prolonged QT-interval.** The U-waves of hypokalemia tend to be most prominent in the precordial leads, as they are here. Hypokalemia may sometimes produce U-waves in the limb leads as well, but often the limb leads simply demonstrate T-wave flattening and/or QT-interval prolongation. Other ECG findings that are typical of hypokalemia include ST-segment depression, as noted in the inferior leads here, and atrial or ventricular ectopy. This patient's serum potassium level was 2.5 mEq/L (normal 3.5–5.3 mEq/L). The U-waves and the ST-segment depression resolved with potassium replacement.

145. **Atrial fibrillation, ventricular rate 180, WPW.** Seven of the first eight QRS complexes occur in a regular pattern and have a narrow QRS morphology. This may represent sinus activity, though the artifact obscures a definite diagnosis. However, the rhythm then becomes irregularly irregular, *very* rapid (with rates approaching >250 beats/minute in some sections), and wide with QRS complex morphologies that vary in width. These three characteristics are typical of atrial fibrillation in the presence of an accessory pathway. Atrial fibrillation that utilizes the

normal His-Purkinje conduction system, in contrast, produces ventricular rates that rarely exceed 180 beats/minute *at any time*, and the morphology of the QRS complexes has much less variation from beat to beat. The distinction between atrial fibrillation with a bundle branch block or non-specific IVCD versus atrial fibrillation with WPW is critical: treatment of the former with AV-nodal blocking medications (e.g. calcium channel blockers, beta blockers, digoxin, amiodarone) is appropriate, whereas treatment of the latter with these medications is deadly. This patient was treated with amiodarone and developed ventricular fibrillation, which fortunately was converted to SR with prompt defibrillation (amiodarone has calcium channel and beta blocking effects and is best avoided in these patients). Procainamide or electrical cardioversion are generally considered the most appropriate management strategies for patients with atrial fibrillation and WPW with rapid ventricular rates.

146. **ST with AV dissociation and third degree AV block, junctional escape rhythm, rate 66, RBBB.** The atrial complexes are subtle but they are regular at a rate of 107 beats/minute. The ventricular rate is also regular. The PR-intervals vary randomly, a characteristic of AV dissociation. There is no evidence that any of the P-waves are conducted to the ventricle, therefore third degree (complete) heart block is diagnosed. The escape rhythm is wide, suggesting a ventricular pacemaker, but the QRS morphology is typical of a RBBB (rsR' in lead V1, wide S-waves in leads I, V5, and V6). The T-wave inversions in the right precordial leads are also typical of (and normal for) RBBB. Therefore, the escape rhythm is diagnosed as a junctional rhythm with RBBB. See figure below.

This figure corresponds to case #146

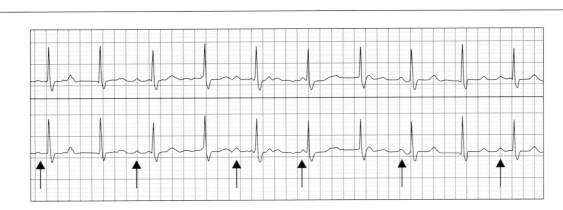

Note the AV dissociation with rapid atrial rate and slower ventricular response. In the setting of AV dissociation and no apparent AV conduction, third degree (complete) heart block is diagnosed. The P-waves (arrows) are seen in this rhythm strip.

147. **ST, rate 109, possible inferior MI of undetermined age, PRWP, T-wave abnormality consistent with inferior and anteroseptal ischemia, consider pulmonary embolism.** Although T-wave inversions are usually considered a sign of cardiac ischemia, acute pulmonary embolism should always be considered as well. Marriott[5] has noted that the simultaneous presence of T-wave inversions in the inferior and anteroseptal leads is highly suggestive of acute pulmonary hypertension, which in emergency medicine usually equates to pulmonary embolism. Kosuge[3] also found that this abnormality was 99% specific for acute pulmonary embolism rather than acute cardiac ischemia. Small q-waves are noted in two of the inferior leads suggestive of a prior inferior MI, and PRWP (defined as an R-wave amplitude <3 mm in lead V3) suggests the possibility of a prior anteroseptal MI. During this patient's workup, he was found to have evidence of prior MIs but no active cardiac ischemia, and bilateral acute pulmonary emboli were diagnosed.

148. **ST, rate 107, acute pericarditis.** Slight STE is present in multiple leads. Potential causes of diffuse STE include acute pericarditis, massive acute MI, benign early repolarization, coronary vasospasm, and LVH. Of these various causes, acute pericarditis is the only one that causes PR-segment depression, a finding noted here in leads I, II, aVF, V5, and V6. The only other ECG abnormality that is considered highly specific for acute pericarditis is PR-segment elevation >2 mm in lead aVR, although in this case lead aVR is not helpful because the PR-segment elevation is not prominent.

This figure corresponds to case #148. PR-segment abnormalities in acute pericarditis

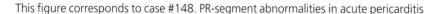

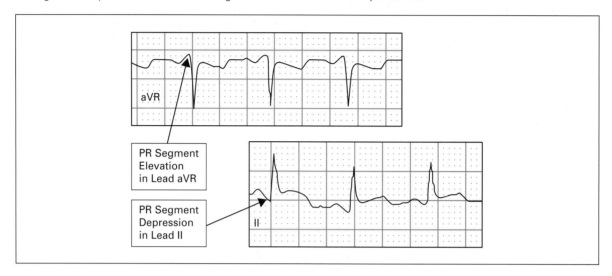

149. **ST, rate 115, low voltage and electrical alternans suggestive of pericardial effusion, lateral ischemia.** Low voltage is diagnosed when the QRS amplitudes in all of the limb leads are <5 mm, or when the QRS amplitudes in all of the precordial leads are <10 mm. The differential diagnosis for low voltage includes large pericardial or pleural effusions, myxedema, end-stage cardiomyopathies, severe chronic obstructive pulmonary disease, severe obesity, infiltrative myocardial diseases, constrictive pericarditis, and prior massive MI. This patient's low voltage was a new finding compared to recent prior ECGs, an important diagnostic point. The most common causes of *new* low voltage are large pericardial effusions and large pleural effusions. The combination of new low voltage, tachycardia, and electrical alternans (best noted in lead V3) is diagnostic of large pericardial effusions. This was confirmed, along with pericardial tamponade, on an echocardiography and was caused by a pericardial metastasis from lung cancer. Lateral T-wave inversions suggest ischemia, although mild T-wave abnormalities and mild ST-segment changes are not uncommon in the setting of large pericardial effusions.

150. **SR, probable acute posterior MI.** ST-segment depression is present in leads V1–V3. This could represent anteroseptal ischemia or an isolated acute posterior MI. The horizontal ST-segment depression and upright T-waves are more suggestive of acute posterior MI; anteroseptal ischemia would more likely produce downsloping ST-segment depression and T-wave inversions. ECG confirmation of acute posterior MI could be obtained by repeating the ECG with posterior-placed leads and finding STE or by performing serial ECGs and noting increasing R-wave amplitudes in leads V1–V3. Increasing R-wave amplitudes in the anteroseptal leads is analogous to Q-waves of the posterior wall. This patient was eventually diagnosed with acute posterior MI, but fibrinolytic administration was significantly delayed because posterior MI was not initially considered.

151. **Probable atrial fibrillation/flutter, ventricular rate 175, bifascicular block (RBBB + LAFB), anterolateral ischemia.** This wide QRS complex rhythm demonstrates periods of regularity and irregularity without obvious P-waves. The irregular section is almost certainly atrial fibrillation. The regular sections could be VT, but VT rarely co-exists with atrial fibrillation. The other possible cause of the regularity is atrial flutter, which is often known to co-exist with atrial fibrillation. When medications were given to slow the heart rate, occasional flutter waves became apparent. QRS prolongation is caused by a bifascicular block (RBBB diagnosed based on rsR' in lead V1, wide S-waves in leads I, V5, and V6; LAFB diagnosed based on rS complexes in lead III and qR complexes in lead aVL). Slight variation in the width of QRS complexes can be caused by the magnitude of the aberrant conduction. Notice, however, that the variation in QRS morphologies is not to the degree seen in cases of atrial fibrillation with WPW (see cases #120 and #145 for comparison). Pronounced J-point depression is noted in the anterolateral leads consistent with ischemia. While a few millimeters of ST-segment depression is typically seen in the right precordial leads in the presence of a RBBB, this "normal" ST-segment depression should not extend into leads V4–V6, nor should the depression be this marked.

This figure corresponds to case #151. Atrial fibrillation/flutter with aberrant intraventricular conduction due to a pre-existing bundle branch block

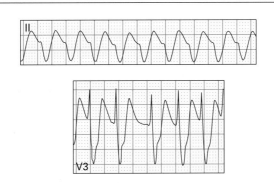

In this case, atrial fibrillation with rapid ventricular response and aberrant ventricular conduction is seen. Note that the degree of variation of QRS complex morphology is negligible. Also, observe that the perceived regularity is present at more rapid rates (lead II) as compared to the relatively slower rates in lead V3.

152. **SR, rate 76, LBBB, ST-segment abnormality consistent with acute ischemia or MI.** Acute MI in this patient with LBBB is suggested based on positive Sgarbossa criteria[1] (described in case #111) in leads aVL, V5, and V6. In each of these leads, STE is present that is concordant with the QRS complexes. Additionally the inferior leads demonstrate concerning findings as well—ST-segment depression is concordant with the terminal deflection of the QRS complexes (note that even though the major portion of the QRS complex in lead II is upright, the *terminal deflection* is downward). Although the presence of concordant ST-segment depression in the inferior leads is not a Sgarbossa criterion, it should still raise concerns of ischemia in patients with LBBB. See figure on p. 182.

153. **SR, rate 97, incomplete RBBB with STE in septal leads suggestive of the Brugada syndrome, left atrial enlargement.** The Brugada syndrome, described in more detail in case #126, is characterized by an incomplete or complete RBBB QRS pattern in the right precordial leads with STE. This patient has convex upward STE, which is more sensitive and specific for the syndrome. Definitive diagnosis is made in the electrophysiology laboratory, whereupon patients are treated with placement of an internal cardioverter-defibrillator. This is the only effective prophylaxis against sudden death (no medications are proven to be effective). This patient was urgently referred

This figure corresponds to case #152. LBBB and acute MI

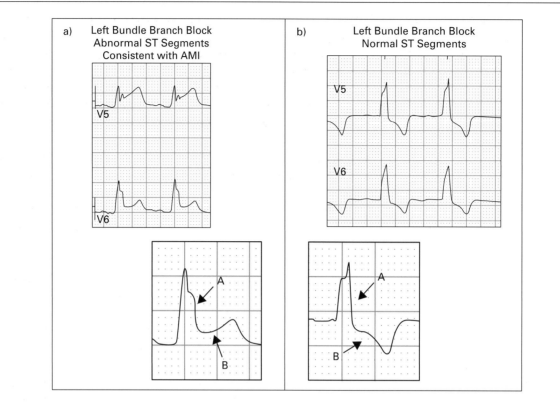

a) Electrocardiographic acute MI is seen in this example. Note that [A], the major terminal portion of the QRS complex, is on the same side of the baseline as [B], the ST-segment. This relationship is abnormal and termed concordant STE, a finding that is very suggestive of acute MI in the presence of LBBB. b) These complexes illustrate the normal, or expected, relationship between the major terminal portion of the QRS complex [A] with the ST-segment [B]. In this example, the QRS complex and ST-segment are located on opposite sides of the baseline, termed appropriate discordance.

for electrophysiologic testing. The diagnosis was confirmed and she received an internal cardioverter-defibrillator. Left atrial enlargement is diagnosed based on a downward terminal deflection of the P-wave in lead V1 with amplitude of at least 1 mm and duration of 40 msec.

154. **ST, acute pericarditis, electrical alternans suggestive of pericardial effusion.** Diffuse STE is present. Diagnostic considerations for this finding should include acute pericarditis, large acute MI, vasospasm, and benign early repolarization. The ECG features suggestive of acute pericarditis are PR-segment depression/ downsloping (subtle) in multiple leads and also the electrical alternans in leads V5–V6. Although the QRS complexes do not demonstrate low voltage, the presence of tachycardia, STE, and electrical alternans are highly suggestive of acute pericarditis with pericardial effusion. Acute pericarditis is the only one of the four entities listed above which would be expected to occur with a pericardial effusion. An echocardiogram confirmed a moderate size effusion. Small upward deflections are noted within the T-waves of the precordial leads. They do not map out with the normal P-waves and therefore do not represent flutter waves. They were assumed to be artifact, and they did not appear on subsequent ECGs.

155. **Probable atrial fibrillation, ventricular rate 45, occasional PVCs, low voltage, non-specific IVCD.** Atrial fibrillation is diagnosed based on the irregularity of the intrinsic complexes and absence of distinct atrial activity. The ventricular response is unusually slow for atrial fibrillation. When atrial fibrillation with a very slow ventricular response is present, the physician should consider several specific diagnostic possibilities: hypothermia, medication toxicity (especially digoxin), sick sinus syndrome, and severe hyperkalemia. This dysrhythmia may also be a pre-terminal rhythm. Because the patient was hypotensive, transcutaneous pacing was attempted but failed to capture. Intravenous atropine was also given without any improvement. By this time, the patient's serum potassium level was reported at 8.4 mEq/L (normal 3.5–5.3 mEq/L). Intravenous calcium and sodium bicarbonate were then administered with prompt return of sinus rhythm and and improvement in the ventricular rate and blood pressure. In retrospect, subtle clues to hyperkalemia were present. The patient has slight QRS complex prolongation and prominent precordial T-waves (albeit not markedly "peaked"). Hyperkalemia is also known to produce unusual bradydysrhythmias, AV blocks, and long pauses between groups of QRS complexes. Severe hyperkalemia usually co-exists with severe metabolic acidosis. Transcutaneouos pacing, atropine, and vasopressors are often ineffective in the setting of severe acidosis, and as a result normal treatments for bradycardia tend to be ineffective if hyperkalemia is responsible. The prudent emergency physician should always consider hyperkalemia in the differential diagnosis for bradycardia, especially if the rhythm appears *particularly* unusual.

156. **SB, rate 49, PRWP, LAFB, T-wave abnormality consistent with Wellens' syndrome.** Wellens' syndrome, first described in 1982,[6] is characterized by an electrocardiographic T-wave abnormality in the mid-precordial leads (leads V2, V3, and sometimes V4 as well). This T-wave pattern was found to be very highly specific for critical stenosis in the proximal LAD artery. These patients are best managed with PCI; medical management alone was found to be associated with a poor short-term outcome. The T-wave pattern can occur in either of two types. In the Type 1 pattern the T-waves are deeply inverted and symmetric. In the Type 2 pattern, the T-waves are biphasic. In neither of the two patterns is ST-segment elevation or depression necessarily present, nor are cardiac biomarkers reliably elevated. Additionally, these patients can be asymptomatic at the time of the ECG recording, i.e. the T-wave abnormality is not dependent on active ischemia. PRWP (R-wave in lead V3 <3mm) and LAFB (leftward axis with qR complexes in leads I and aVL and rS complexes in lead III) are present. After an unremarkable laboratory workup in the ED this patient was discharged. The ECG was interpreted as having a "non-specific" T-wave abnormality. On the contrary, the T-wave abnormality was *very* specific and predicted the eventual outcome: her symptoms recurred several days later, at which time she was diagnosed with an acute anterior MI. She was taken for PCI and found to have a 100% LAD occlusion.

157. **SR with second degree AV block type 2 (Mobitz II), rate 40, RBBB.** The atrial rate is 73, and there are frequent non-conducted P-waves that result in an overall bradycardic ventricular rate. A second degree AV block is present mostly with a 2:1 conduction ratio (two P-waves for every one QRS). When 2:1 conduction occurs, it is impossible to determine with certainty whether the rhythm is Mobitz I or Mobitz II. In this case, however, 3:2 conduction occurs in one portion of the rhythm strip: in the 5th–6th ventricular beats. In this area, the PR-interval remains constant. This confirms the diagnosis of Mobitz II.

158. **ST with second degree AV block and 2:1 conduction, rate 90, occasional aberrant ventricular conduction.** This rhythm was misinterpreted as simply sinus rhythm with a rate of 90. However, on close inspection one notices that the T-waves have a slightly unusual morphology. Although they are not tall, they have a slightly "peaked" appearance in some leads, and in lead III there is slight deformity noted within the T-wave (a small secondary upward deflection). While large peaked T-waves are characteristic of hyperkalemia, smaller peaked T-waves and T-waves with deformities or secondary deflections should always raise consideration of buried, or partially hidden, atrial activity. In this case, the peaked areas on the T-waves do in fact map out with the P-waves. These are buried atrial beats. The atrial rate, therefore, is actually 180 with second degree block and 2:1

conduction (when second degree block occurs with 2:1 conduction, specific designation of Mobitz I or Mobitz II is deferred). Because the unusual T-wave morphology here was not closely scrutinized, this patient was not admitted to a critical care bed, nor was any consideration given to possible pacemaker placement. On the night of admission, the patient progressed to third degree heart block, had a cardiac arrest, and died. At that point, this originally ECG was more closely scrutinized and the mistake was realized. This ECG also demonstrates slight variation in QRS complex morphology between some beats, the result of slight aberrancy in ventricular conduction. However the QRS complexes remain of normal duration and do not meet criteria for a bundle branch block or fascicular block.

159. **SB, ventricular rate 100, frequent PVCs in a pattern of ventricular bigeminy, acute inferior MI.** The sinus rate appears to be approximately 50 beats/minute, though it is uncertain if additional P-waves are obscured by the PVCs. Despite the presence of the PVCs, STE is seen in the inferior leads. The ST-segment depression in the anteroseptal leads is downsloping and these leads do not have prominent R-waves, so this ST-segment depression is suspected to represent reciprocal change and *not* concurrent posterior MI. Reciprocal ST-segment depression is also noted in lateral leads. This patient was treated with beta blocking medications for the ventricular ectopy and underwent a successful PCI. See figure below.

This figure corresponds to case #159. R-on-T PVC with degeneration to malignant ventricular dysrhythmia

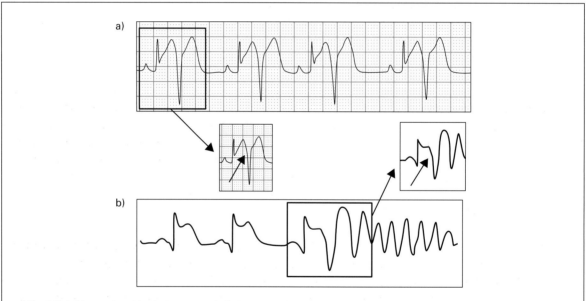

a) Lead II rhythm strip with obvious acute inferior wall MI and ventricular bigeminy with R-on-T pattern. This rhythm is somewhat dangerous in that the R-wave, delivered on an electrically vulnerable period of the P-QRS-T cycle, can precipitate ventricular tachycardia or fibrillation. The insert demonstrates the R-wave falling on the T-wave (arrow) of the sinus beat. b) The R-on-T event degenerates into a malignant ventricular dysrhythmia (from a different patient). Note the R-wave again falling on the T-wave (arrow) resulting in a pulseless cardiac arrest.

160. **ST, rate 130, LBBB.** The rhythm is a regular wide QRS complex tachycardia. As is often the case, P-waves are best noted in lead V1. Failure to recognize these P-waves could easily result in misdiagnosis of the rhythm as VT and lead to unnecessary and potentially harmful therapies, e.g. cardioversion or antidysrhythmics. The ECG demonstrates the normal, expected discordance in LBBB between the QRS complexes and ST-segments. The

abrupt transition in R-wave size between leads V5 to V6 is likely the result of rightward misplacement of lead V5. This patient had pneumonia and dehydration. His heart rate improved with intravenous fluids.

161. **SB, ventricular rate 105, frequent PVCs, acute inferior-posterior MI.** The intrinsic sinus P-waves appear at a rate of approximately 48 beats/minute, though it is uncertain if additional P-waves are obscured by PVCs. The PVCs appear mostly in a pattern of bigeminy, though consecutive PVCs appear just after the half-way point of the ECG. The intrinsic beats have associated STE in the inferior leads, consistent with an acute inferior MI. In the right precordial leads, there is also evidence of acute posterior MI: ST-segment depression, tall R-waves, and upright T-waves. Much like case #159, this patient was treated with beta blocking medications for the ventricular ectopy and underwent a successful PCI for a 100% occluded right coronary artery.

162. **Accelerated idioventricular rhythm, rate 114.** The rhythm is a regular wide QRS complex tachycardia without obvious sinus activity. The first assumption in this scenario should always be VT. However, the diagnosis of VT should be reserved for patients with a ventricular rate of ≥120 beats/minute. Normal ventricular escape rhythms (or "idioventricular" rhythms) are 20–40 beats/minute. When the rhythm is 40–120 beats/minute, it is referred to as an *accelerated* idioventricular rhythm (AIVR). This rhythm is commonly seen in acute MI patients who reperfuse either spontaneously or through medical therapy (e.g. fibrinolytics). As a result, it is often referred to in this setting as a "reperfusion dysrhythmia," although it may occur in non-MI settings as well. The rhythm itself should not produce hemodynamic instability and therefore does not warrant suppression with antidysrhythmics such as lidocaine, amiodarone, or procainamide. In fact, use of these medications can be deadly, as the rhythm converts to asystole. Instead, observation is warranted during which the dysrhythmia spontaneously resolves, usually within minutes. Ventricular antidysrhythmics should be reserved for patients with VT—primary ventricular rhythms ≥120 beats/minute. This patient converted to sinus rhythm after several minutes without receiving any medications.

163. **Atrial flutter with 2:1 AV conduction, ventricular rate 150, inferior and possible lateral MI of undetermined age.** This patient was originally diagnosed as having ST based on what appear to be normal P-waves in some of the leads. The patient was treated with two liters of intravenous fluids under the assumption that he was dehydrated. When the heart rate didn't improve with fluids, several hours later, the proper diagnosis was realized. As discussed in prior cases, lead V1 often provides the best view of atrial activity. Whenever the ventricular rate is 150 ± 20 beats/minute all 12 leads, especially lead V1, should be closely examined for evidence of atrial flutter. Q-waves are present in the inferior leads indicating prior inferior MI. Q-waves in lead V6 are also present, indicating possible prior lateral MI.

164. **Atrial fibrillation, ventricular rate 147, LBBB, ST-segment abnormality consistent with acute ischemia or MI.** Acute MI in this patient with LBBB is suggested based on positive Sgarbossa criteria[1] (described in case #111) in lead V3. The normal ST-segment in lead V3 in a patient with LBBB is elevated up to 5 mm, whereas this patient has pronounced concordant ST-segment depression. Several other leads demonstrate findings that, although not meeting Sgarbossa criteria, are nevertheless concerning: (1) leads II, aVF, and V4 demonstrate ST-segment depression that is concordant with the terminal deflection of the QRS complexes; and (2) the ST-segments in leads V5–V6 demonstrate *excessive* discordance (≥5 mm in the opposite direction) to the terminal deflection of the QRS complex. This patient was sent for emergent PCI and was found to have significant occlusions of both the LMCA as well as the RCA. Despite aggressive management she died.

165. **SR with first degree AV block, acute inferior MI, probable acute right ventricular MI, probable acute posterior MI, LVH.** First degree AV block is diagnosed based on the PR-interval ≥200 msec. STE is present in the inferior leads consistent with acute inferior MI. Patients with acute inferior MI are at risk for extension of the infarct to the right ventricle and/or the posterior wall. The use of additional leads placed on the right chest and

the left mid back area can be helpful in diagnosing right ventricular and posterior infarct, respectively (see figure below). However, this standard 12-lead ECG provides clues to these diagnoses already. In the presence of an acute inferior MI, right ventricular extension is strongly suggested when the magnitude of the STE in lead III is much greater than the magnitude of the STE in lead II. Essentially, lead III on the standard ECG provides a "glance" at the right ventricle. In this case, there is 4 mm of STE in lead III compared to 2.5 mm of STE in lead II. A right-sided ECG was performed and demonstrated STE in the right-sided leads, confirming the presence of acute right ventricular MI. Acute posterior MI is strongly suggested based on the presence of ST-segment depression, tall R-waves, and upright T-waves in the right precordial leads. Acute posterior MI was confirmed by echocardiography. A repeat ECG performed two days later showed residual tall R-waves in these leads. Tall R-waves in leads V1–V3 can be thought of as the "Q-waves of the posterior wall." Leftward axis is present. The usual causes of leftward axis include LAFB, LBBB, inferior MI (if large Q-waves are present), LVH, ventricular ectopy, paced beats, and WPW. The leftward axis is caused by LVH in this case, diagnosed based on R-waves in lead aVL >11 mm in height.

This figure corresponds to case #165

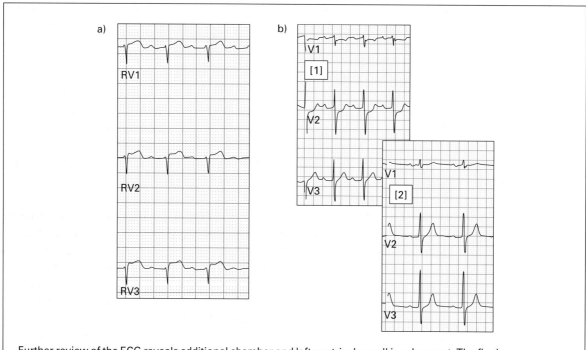

Further review of the ECG reveals additional chamber and left ventricular wall involvement. The final electrocardiographic diagnosis is an inferior-posterior MI with right ventricular (RV) infarction. a) STE in leads RV1–RV3, indicating an infarction of the RV. b) [1] ECG at presentation with acute posterior wall MI present. Note the prominent R-waves in leads V2 and V3 coupled with the ST-segment depression and upright T-waves. [2] ECG from several days after the event demonstrating prominent R-waves in leads V1–V3, indicating a completed posterior wall infarction. Acutely, on presentation, the posterior wall MI was manifested by the prominent R-waves, ST-segment depression, and upright T-waves in leads V1–V3.

166. **SR with premature AV junctional complexes (PJCs) in a pattern of junctional trigeminy, rate 67, WPW, intermittent RBBB, inferolateral ischemia.** The intrinsic beats in the rhythm strip are the shorter QRS complexes that are preceded by P-waves. They occur at a rate of 67 beats/minute. The PR-interval that precedes these

complexes is short (<120 msec). The two major causes of a short PR-interval are WPW and AV junctional beats. WPW is confirmed in these complexes by the presence of delta waves (slurred upstroke of the QRS complexes), best seen in the lateral leads. WPW is responsible for the leftward axis as well as the Q-waves in the inferior leads—WPW often mimics inferior MI in this way. Every third QRS complex is a premature complex. These are narrow complexes and they are associated with either short PR-intervals (the first premature beat) or retro-grade P-waves. This is characteristic of QRS complexes that are originating in the AV junction, thus the de-signation of premature junctional complexes. These PJCs have an rSr' pattern in V1, the result of conduction with an incomplete RBBB. T-wave inversions consistent with ischemia are noted in the inferior leads and non-specific T-waves are noted with slight ST-segment depression in the lateral leads, consistent with inferolateral ischemia.

167. **ST, rate 157, probable severe hyperkalemia.** There appear to be P-waves associated with the QRS com-plexes, best seen again in leads V1 and V2. With a rhythm diagnosis of ST, there are two major possibilities for the unusual morphology of the QRS complexes: (1) this patient is having an acute inferior-anterior MI with massive STE that is giving the *appearance* of QRS complex prolongation; or (2) there is marked prolongation of the QRS complex, likely the result of a metabolic abnormality such as hyperkalemia or the result of toxicity from a sodium channel blocking drug. Favoring the latter possibility is the presence of a rightward axis. Besides hyperkalemia and sodium channel blocking medication toxicity, conditions that produce a rightward axis include old lateral MI (if large Q-waves are present), LPFB, RVH, acute (e.g. pulmonary embolism) or chronic (e.g. emphysema) pulmonary disease, and ventricular ectopy. However, the ECG does not demonstrate diagnostic criteria for any of these other conditions. Absence of Q-waves in lateral leads V5–V6 decreases the possibility that this rightward axis is attributable to MI. Sodium channel blocker toxicity also is unlikely given the absence of wide S-waves all of the lateral leads. In this ECG, leads V5 and V6 lack the wide S-waves that are typical of significant toxicity (see case #125 for comparison). Hyperkalemia remains the most probable diagnosis. The ECG was originally diagnosed as large acute MI, but the patient did prove to have hyperkalemia. The serum potassium level was 8.7 mEq/L (normal 3.5–5.3 mEq/L).

168. **SB with first degree AV block, rate 57, blocked PACs, RBBB, inferior and anteroseptal MI of undeter-mined age, LVH.** The rhythm was originally misdiagnosed as second degree AV block (specifically, Mobitz II) and there was some discussion about placement of a pacemaker in this patient before the correct diagnosis was finally made. The misdiagnosis occurred because of the presence of non-conducted P-waves. The 2nd and 7th P-waves on the rhythm strip are non-conducted and followed by a pause. However, the diagnosis of second degree AV block (either Mobitz I or Mobitz II) requires a second criterion: the P-P intervals must be relatively constant. In this particular case, the 2nd and 7th P-waves arrive early (and have a slightly different morphology than the other P-waves). These are PACs. When PACs occur too early in the cycle, during ventricular repolarization, they may be conducted aberrantly (e.g. with a RBBB) or they may not be conducted at all to the ventricle. In the latter case, these non-conducted or "blocked" PACs are then simply followed by a pause during which time the sinus node "resets" and then continues normal activity. These PACs in themselves are benign, though they may simply cause the patient to experience some palpitations. They are often caused by mild electrolyte abnormalities (slight hypokalemia in this case), medications, caffeine, over-the-counter sympathomimetics (e.g. cold medications), etc. However, blocked PACs often result in a misdiagnosis of Mobitz II if the treating physician does not closely exam-ine the P-P intervals. The ECG also demonstrates evidence of a RBBB with typical ST-segment/T-wave abnormali-ties in leads V1–V3. A prior anteroseptal MI is diagnosed based on the q-waves in the right precordial leads, although small, combined with the loss of normal R-waves (loss of normal anterior forces) in leads V4–V6. Similarly, prior inferior MI is diagnosed based on the loss of R-waves in the inferior leads. LVH is diagnosed based on R-waves in lead aVL >11 mm.

169. **SR with AV dissociation and third degree AV block, AV junctional escape rhythm, rate 52, acute inferior-posterior MI, probable acute right ventricular MI.** The P-waves are very subtle, best seen in the lead II rhythm strip at a rate of 88 beats/minute. Atrial and ventricular activity are independent (AV dissociation) and there does not appear to be any P-waves that are conducted (third degree AV block). The escape rhythm demonstrates narrow QRS complexes at a rate typical for the AV junction. STE with early q-wave formation is present in the inferior leads consistent with acute MI. Reciprocal ST-segment depression is present in leads I and aVL. ST-segment depression is present in leads V2–V3 could represent reciprocal change or acute posterior MI. The presence of upright T-waves in these leads and tall R-waves in all three right precordial leads strongly favors acute posterior MI rather than reciprocal change. Acute right ventricular MI is suggested by the presence of STE in lead III significantly greater in magnitude than the STE in lead II (3 mm versus 1 mm). A repeat ECG with right precordial leads confirmed acute right ventricular MI (see figure below). The diagnosis of right ventricular MI is important in that it mandates a change in normal MI management: preload-reducing medications (e.g. nitrates) must be used with great caution, and aggressive use of intravenous fluids is often needed to maintain the blood pressure. This patient developed pronounced hypotension prior to arrival when the prehospital care providers administered nitroglycerin. His blood pressure improved only after a liter of intravenous fluids had been administered.

This figure corresponds to case #169

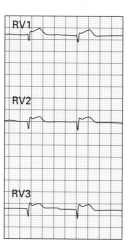

STE in the right-sided leads—RV infarction. Minimal STE, in the appropriate clinical setting (inferior wall MI with hypotension), should prompt the consideration of an RV MI. Recall that the right ventricular myocardium is composed of relatively less muscle mass; thus, a current of injury will generate a lower magnitude of STE.

170. **SR, rate 83, left atrial enlargement (LAE), prolonged QT-interval, suspected hypocalcemia.** The QT-interval prolongation (QT is 472 msec but QTc is 554 msec) provides the main diagnostic clue. In almost all causes of QT-interval prolongation, the QT-interval is prolonged due primarily to prolongation of the T-wave. However, in this case the T-wave appears normal in size. Instead the QT-interval is prolonged due to prolongation of the *ST-*

segment. In the differential diagnosis of a prolonged QT-interval (hypokalemia, hypomagnesemia, hypocalcemia, acute myocardial ischemia, elevated intracranial pressure, sodium channel blocking medications, hypothermia, and congenital prolonged QT-interval), only two entities primarily prolong the ST-segment: hypocalcemia and hypothermia. Hypothermia less likely given the absence of bradycardia. This patient did in fact have hypocalcemia (5.1 mg/dL; normal 8.8–10.2 mg/dL) due to hypoparathyroidism. LAE is diagnosed when the P-wave is notched and has a duration >110 msec in any of the leads; and when the downward terminal deflection of the P-wave in lead V1 has an amplitude ≥1 mm and duration ≥40 msec.

171. **Ectopic atrial tachycardia with variable AV block, ventricular rate 55, occasional PVCs, anteroseptal MI of undetermined age, probable inferior MI of undetermined age, lateral ischemia; rhythm suggestive of digoxin toxicity.** Subtle atrial activity (best seen in lead V1) is noted at a rate of 167 beats/minute, though the presence of inverted P-waves in lead I, and the presence of upright P-waves in aVR, excludes a sinus node origin. The ventricular response is slow and variable in ratio. Atrial tachycardia with variable AV block and slow ventricular response is a common dysrhythmia associated with digoxin toxicity. PVCs are also present and, although not specific for digoxin toxicity, are the most common finding in the presence of digoxin toxicity. This patient's serum digoxin level was 4.2 ng/mL (normal 0.5–2.2 ng/mL). Q-waves present in leads V1–V4 indicate prior anteroseptal MI, and Q-waves present in two of the three inferior leads indicate *probable* inferior MI. T-wave inversions in leads I, aVL, and V6 indicate lateral ischemia.

172. **ST with second degree AV block type 1 (Wenckebach, Mobitz I), rate 68, lateral ischemia.** The sinus rate is 107 beats/minute. The rhythm is challenging to interpret because the PR-intervals are markedly prolonged and the AV conduction ratios vary—2:1 ratio is present in the early portion of the rhythm strip, followed by a 4:3 section, then 3:2 conduction. Mobitz I is diagnosed based on PR-interval prolongation preceding the non-conducted P-waves. T-wave inversions consistent with ischemia are present in the lateral leads.

173. **ST, rate 126, incomplete RBBB with STE in septal leads suggestive of the Brugada syndrome, LAFB, diffuse ischemia.** The Brugada syndrome is an electrophysiological phenomenon associated with sudden cardiac arrest in patients with structurally normal hearts. It is now believed to be responsible for approximately 4% of all sudden deaths and 20% of all sudden deaths in patients without structural heart disease,[7] highlighting the need for all emergency physicians to become aware of the condition. The characteristic ECG finding is an incomplete or complete RBBB pattern with STE in leads V1–V2 (sometimes extending to lead V3) in the resting state. The STE is most commonly convex upwards or straight (as in this case), although the STE less often can be concave upwards instead. Usually there are no reciprocal ST-segment changes as found in acute MI. In this case, however, there are leads with ST-segment depression, likely the result of post-arrest ischemia. This patient survived because of prompt chest compressions by a bystander. The diagnosis was confirmed on electrophysiologic testing and an internal cardioverter-defibrillator, the only effective therapy, was placed.

174. **Atrial flutter with 2:1 AV conduction, ventricular rate 143.** This rhythm was originally diagnosed as ST. The patient was treated with two liters of intravenous fluids under the assumption that ST was caused by dehydration. The fluids did not improve her heart rate, and it was not until she developed hypoxia from heart failure that the misdiagnosis was realized. Whenever the ventricular rate is 150 ± 20 beats/minute, it is imperative to closely examine all 12 leads for evidence of atrial flutter. Lack of this scrutiny is likely the reason that atrial flutter is the most frequently misdiagnosed tachydysrhythmia. In this case, inverted flutter waves are present in the inferior leads, and upright flutter waves are found in the septal leads (some of the flutter waves are "buried" within the T-waves in lead V1). Because our eyes are more accustomed to detecting upright atrial waves than inverted ones, the inverted flutter waves are easily overlooked or discounted as artifact, as they were initially in this case. The authors recommend a simple maneuver to increase the yield in detecting flutter waves: turn the ECG upside

down and re-examine the inferior leads, as described in cases #116 and #132. When the ECG is inverted, flutter waves in lead II at a rate of 286 beats/minute suddenly appear more prominent to the eyes.

175. **ST with second degree AV block type 2 (Mobitz II), rate 83, frequent PJCs and PVCs, anterior ischemia.** This is a difficult ECG rhythm on first glance because of the frequency of ectopic beats. However, the rhythm can be broken down into parts to clarify the diagnosis. See figure below.

This figure corresponds to case #175. Second degree AV block type 2 with frequent premature supraventricular and ventricular beats

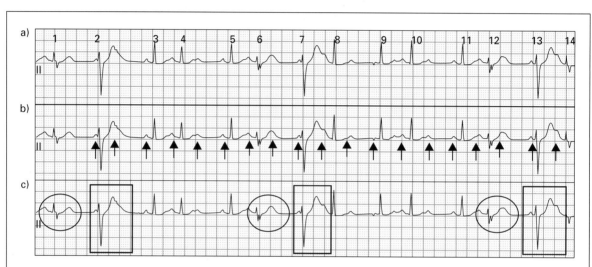

a) The first two QRS complexes appear abnormal. The third QRS complex appears to be the first one that is conducted from a preceding P-wave. b) From that point forward, P-waves clearly appear at a rate of 128/minute and continue throughout the rhythm. Some P-waves are non-conducted, indicating a second degree AV block. The PR-intervals in the beats that *are* conducted (the narrow upright QRS complexes) all remain constant in duration; therefore, Mobitz II is diagnosed. The remaining complexes are simply ectopic beats. c) The 1st, 6th, 12th, and 14th complexes (circled) are wide (QRS duration >120 msec) and not preceded by P-waves, therefore they are presumed to be PVCs. The 2nd, 7th, and 13th complexes (in rectangles) are <120 msec and are therefore likely supraventricular in origin. Each of these is preceded by a sinus P-wave, but the PR-interval in these complexes to too short (<120 msec) to be a conducted atrial beat, therefore they are presumed to be PJCs.

176. **Atrial tachycardia with second degree AV block type 1 (Wenckebach, Mobitz I), 3:2 AV conduction, rate 95, anteroseptal MI of undetermined age.** Because of the significant baseline artifact and irregularity in the rhythm, this patient was misdiagnosed as having atrial fibrillation and placed on anticoagulant medications. This proved to be unnecessary, however. Although the rhythm is irregular, close inspection reveals that it is actually *regularly* irregular, ruling out atrial fibrillation. The two common causes of a regularly irregular rhythm are second degree AV block and ectopic beats that occur regularly (e.g. bigeminy, trigeminy, etc.). In this particular case, close inspection reveals P-waves in some leads (best seen in leads I and V2) at a rate of 143 beats/minute. The accompanying figure on p. 191 highlights the P-waves in lead I and their association to the QRS complexes. There is a gradual lengthening of the PR-interval, and every third P-wave is non-conducted—Mobitz I rhythm in a 3:2 AV conduction ratio is diagnosed. Sinus tachycardia cannot formally be diagnosed because of the artifact, therefore the rhythm is simply referred to as an atrial tachycardia. Q-waves are noted in lead V2, and PRWP is present, consistent with a prior anteroseptal MI. In contrast to atrial flutter, which is considered the most underdiagnosed

tachydysrhythmia, atrial fibrillation is the most overdiagnosed tachydysrhythmia. Overdiagnosis often occurs because of failure to recognize subtle regularity within the overall rhythm. Before diagnosis of atrial fibrillation, the physician should be certain that the ventricular response is truly *irregularly* irregular.

This figure corresponds to case #176. Atrial tachycardia with second degree AV block type 1

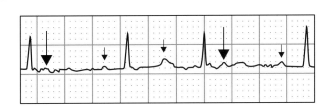

Note the P-waves in this lead I rhythm strip; the small arrows indicate P waves of conducted atrial beats while the large arrows indicated non-conducted P-waves.

177. **Accelerated AV junctional tachycardia, rate 75, frequent PJCs occurring in a pattern of junctional trigeminy.** This case should be compared and contrasted to case #176. The rhythm was once again initially misdiagnosed as atrial fibrillation because of the irregularity. This rhythm, however, is another example of a *regularly* irregular rhythm. In contrast to case #176 where second degree AV block accounted for the regular irregularity, this is a case where regularly-occurring premature complexes are responsible. The underlying rhythm consists of narrow QRS complexes without preceding P-waves—a junctional rhythm. Because the rate is greater than the normal intrinsic rate of the AV junction (40–60 beats/minute), the rhythm is referred to as an *accelerated* AV junctional rhythm. Every third QRS complex (3rd, 6th, 9th, and 12th) occurs early, is narrow, and is not preceded by P-waves. Therefore, these are PJCs occurring in a pattern of junctional trigeminy. This patient's rhythm converted back to SR after a short period of observation. The medication she took was never discovered.

178. **SB, rate 50, LVH, inverted U-waves in lateral leads suggestive of ischemia.** Inverted U-waves are present in the lateral precordial leads (see figure on p. 192). Defined as small negative deflections of even 0.5 mm just after the T-wave, inverted U-waves may be the only sign and a very specific sign of ischemia.[8–10] They tend to occur in the lateral leads and are associated with LAD artery or LMCA occlusion.[10] These U-waves may appear in the resting state or during ischemia symptoms. LVH is diagnosed based on the sum of the amplitudes of the R-wave in lead V5 + S-wave in lead V1 > 35 mm.

179. **SR with AV dissociation and third degree AV block, accelerated AV junctional escape rhythm, rate 83, prominent T-waves suggestive of hyperkalemia.** P-waves are present at a rate of 97 beats/minute. The QRS complexes, however, appear at a rate of 83 beats/minute, indicating AV dissociation. The QRS complexes are narrow (<120 msec) indicating an AV junctional escape rhythm. The rate is faster than the intrinsic rate of the AV junction (40–60 beats/minute), therefore it is referred to as an *accelerated* junctional rhythm. The escape rhythm is completely regular without evidence of conduction of any P-waves so this also represents third degree (complete) heart block. Prominent, "peaked" T-waves appear in the precordial leads suggestive of hyperkalemia. The serum potassium was, in fact, 7.1 mEq/L (normal 3.5–5.3 mEq/L). Hyperkalemia is well-known to produce rhythm disturbances, including atrial or ventricular tachydysrhythmias or bradydysrhythmias and AV blocks. This patient's rhythm converted back to SR after administration of calcium and sodium bicarbonate.

This figure corresponds to case #178

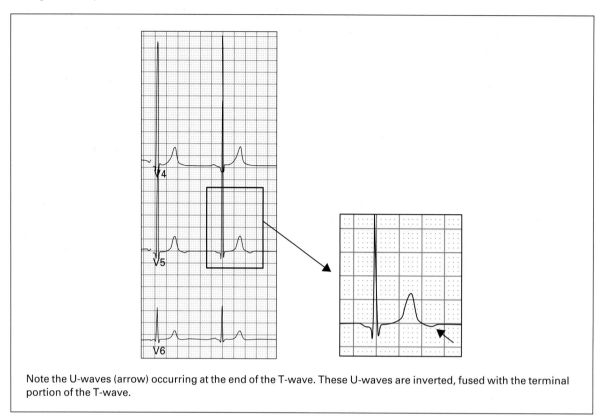

Note the U-waves (arrow) occurring at the end of the T-wave. These U-waves are inverted, fused with the terminal portion of the T-wave.

180. **SR with AV dissociation, AV junctional escape rhythm with RBBB, rate 44, occasional capture beats, inferior and lateral ischemia.** Sinus P-waves appear at a rate of 71 beats/minute but are frequently non-conducted. An escape rhythm occurs at a rate of approximately 40 beats/minute and with a RBBB morphology (see 5th and 6th QRS complexes). These represent an AV junctional rhythm. However, three of the QRS complexes (2nd, 4th, and 7th) occur early, have a slightly different morphology, and are preceded by P-waves with a relatively normal PR-interval (mild first degree block only). These three complexes are the result of conducted P-waves, or "capture beats." In contrast, the other QRS complexes are presumed to be escape beats because they are not preceded by P-waves that could be conducted (the third QRS complex is preceded by a PR-interval that is too short to be conducted; the 1st, 5th, and 6th QRS complexes are preceded by PR-intervals that are too long to be conducted). This is an example of AV dissociation *without* third degree (complete) heart block. Third degree heart block is excluded whenever there is evidence that any of the P-waves are conducted. ST-segment depression in the inferior leads and T-wave inversions in the lateral leads suggests inferior and lateral ischemia.

181. **SR with AV dissociation, ventricular escape rhythm, rate 38, occasional capture beats, lateral ischemia.** This case should reinforce the concepts in case #180. Sinus P-waves appear at a rate of 70 beats/minute but many are non-conducted. A wide QRS complex, ventricular escape rhythm occurs at a rate of 38 beats/minute. A ventricular origin of these complexes is confirmed by the taller "left rabbit ear" in the QRS complexes of lead V1 (compare to the QRS morphology of the RBBB in case #180). The 3rd and 6th QRS complexes occur early in the rhythm and are preceded by P-waves with a relatively normal PR-interval. These two complexes are capture beats, and indicate once again that AV dissociation without complete heart block is present. T-wave inversions following ventricular beats is expected, but the T-wave inversions in the conducted beats indicates ischemia.

182. **SB with first degree AV block, rate 45, blocked PAC, PRWP, possible anteroseptal and inferior MI of undetermined age, low voltage, non-specific IVCD.** This patient's ECG is notable for bradycardia with a profound first degree AV block which was due to the new medication. The rhythm, however, was initially misdiagnosed as a second degree AV block type 2 (Mobitz II) because of the non-conducted P-wave in the mid-portion of the rhythm strip (see figure below). However, the diagnosis of second degree AV block requires that the P-waves occur in a regular rhythm, including the non-conducted P-wave. In this case, however, the non-conducted P-wave occurs early: it is simply a PAC. When PACs occur too early in the cycle, during ventricular repolarization, they may not be conducted at all to the ventricle. These non-conducted or "blocked" PACs are then simply followed by a pause during which time the sinus node "resets" and then continues normal activity. These PACs in themselves are benign, but they often result in a misdiagnosis of Mobitz II if the treating physician does not closely examine the P-P intervals. PRWP is present, indicating possible prior anteroseptal MI. Small q-waves are present in two of the three inferior leads. Although they are less than 40 msec in duration, they are *relatively* large in comparison to the QRS complex and therefore considered possible indication of a prior inferior MI. Low voltage is diagnosed based on QRS complex amplitudes <5 mm in all of the limb leads. The differential diagnosis for low voltage includes myxedema, large pericardial or pleural effusions, end-stage cardiomyopathy, severe chronic obstructive pulmonary disease, severe obesity, infiltrative myocardial diseases, constrictive pericarditis, and prior massive MI. Low voltage in this case was attributed to the patient's cardiomyopathy.

This figure corresponds to case #182

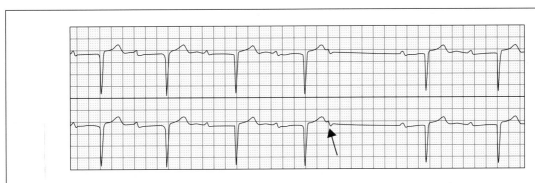

Note the non-conducted PAC—the single P-wave partially obscured by the T-wave (arrow).

183. **ST, rate 105, inferior and anterior ischemia, T-wave abnormality consistent with inferior and anteroseptal ischemia, consider pulmonary embolism.** T-wave inversions are a common finding in cases of large pulmonary emboli, and literature indicates that simultaneous T-wave inversions in the inferior and anteroseptal leads are very specific for acute pulmonary embolism.[3,5] This patient was found to have two large pulmonary emboli.

184. **ST, rate 120, frequent PVCs, diffuse ischemia, prolonged QT-interval.** Diffuse ST-segment depression is present suggesting ischemia. Additionally, marked QT-interval prolongation is present (QT = 410 msec, QTc = 580 msec). The differential diagnosis of QT-interval prolongation includes myocardial ischemia, but the prolongation tends to be more mild; this degree of QT-interval prolongation is unusual for myocardial ischemia and should prompt consideration of other conditions. Other potential causes of QT-interval prolongation include hypokalemia, hypomagnesemia, hypocalcemia, elevated intracranial pressure, drugs with sodium channel blocking effects, hypothermia, and congenital prolonged QT syndrome. During the workup this patient was found to have severe hypokalemia—the serum potassium level was 2.1 mEq/L (normal 3.5–5.3 mEq/L). After supplemental

potassium was administered and the serum level was corrected, the ST-segment depression, PVCs, and QT-interval prolongation all resolved. The other two abnormalities associated with hypokalemia, though not prominent in this case, are U-waves and T-wave flattening.

185. **ST, rate 112, non-specific IVCD, consider sodium-channel blocking drug toxicity or overdose.** A rightward axis is present. The differential diagnosis for rightward axis includes LPFB, lateral MI (due to large Q-waves), RVH, acute (e.g. pulmonary embolism) and chronic (e.g. emphysema) lung disease, sodium-channel blocking drug toxicity (e.g. cyclic antidepressants), and misplaced leads. Normal or slender adults with a horizontally positioned heart can also demonstrate a rightward QRS axis. Amongst these possibilities, only three are associated with widening of the QRS complex: ventricular ectopy, hyperkalemia, and overdoses of sodium-channel blocking drugs. Ventricular ectopy can quickly be ruled out, as the rhythm is ST. Hyperkalemia is unlikely as well, given the absence of prominent T-waves. The ECG as well as the history of delirium are consistent with drug toxicity or overdose. This patient's ECG demonstrates another finding that is typical of cyclic antidepressant toxicity—a tall R-wave in lead aVR. This patient did, in fact, attempt suicide by ingesting tricyclic antidepressant medications. The patient received intravenous boluses of sodium bicarbonate which resulted in prompt narrowing of the QRS complex, reduction in height of the R-wave in lead aVR, and normalization of the axis.

This figure corresponds to case #185. Sodium-channel blocking medication toxicity

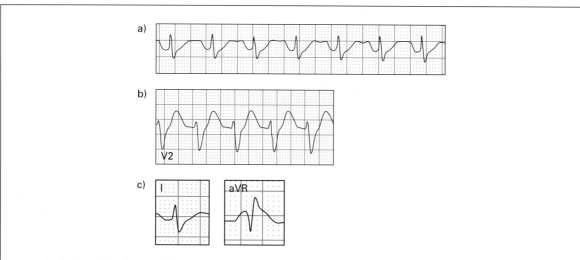

Note the three classic abnormalities seen in the patient with tricyclic antidepressant (TCA) overdose. These findings, when encountered individually, are suggestive; when seen together in a patient with any mental status abnormality, are very strongly suggestive of TCA ingestion. a) Sinus tachycardia. b) Wide QRS complex. c) Prominent S-wave in lead I and R′ wave in lead aVR.

186. **ST, rate 106, diffuse ischemia.** The ECG was initially interpreted as acute pericarditis. Many of the leads demonstrate apparent PR-segment downsloping that is often considered diagnostic of this condition. Additionally, when the PR-segment is used as the baseline or isoelectric segment of the ECG, it appears that there is ST-segment elevation in those same leads. However, when the PR-segment appears to slope downwards or be frankly depressed, it *should not* be used as the baseline. Rather, it is the T-P segment that represents the baseline or isoelectric segment of the ECG. With this in mind, it becomes obvious that the ECG actually does not demonstrate STE, but rather ST-segment depression in many leads (see figure opposite), and therefore acute pericarditis is excluded. PR-segment depression can be caused by other entities besides acute pericarditis—atrial infarction, abnormal

atrial repolarization, etc. PR-segment depression or downsloping is specific for acute pericarditis *only in the setting of STE*. This patient was initially treated for acute pericarditis, but when cardiac biomarkers results were obtained and were markedly positive, she was taken for PCI and found to have diffuse coronary occlusions. She received two stents and fortunately did well despite the delay in proper diagnosis.

This figure corresponds to case #186

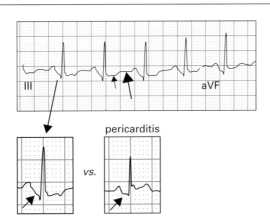

The PR-segment is depressed in this patient initially misdiagnosed with pericarditis. The PR-segment, however, is depressed in a downsloping morphology—a finding which is not necessarily consistent with pericarditis. The ST-segment is depressed, as indicated by the small arrow, when compared to the baseline (large arrow), another finding that excludes the diagnosis of acute pericarditis. Note the insert demonstrating PR-segment depression in pericarditis, which is horizontally depressed, with co-existing ST segment elevation.

187. **SR, rate 95, incomplete RBBB with STE in septal leads suggestive of the Brugada syndrome.** The Brugada syndrome has been described in several prior cases. This case demonstrates the "coved" or convex-upwards type of STE in leads V1–V2 that is most specific for the syndrome. Patients with the Brugada syndrome have a propensity to develop spontaneous episodes of polymorphic (most common) or monomorphic VT. If bystanders or healthcare workers are not immediately available to intervene, the rhythm frequently degenerates into ventricular fibrillation and cardiac arrest results. If the VT spontaneously aborts, however, patients typically present to the healthcare provider describing symptoms of the dysrhythmia—usually palpitations, lightheadedness, or syncope. Those are the patients for whom the healthcare provider must be familiar with the ECG findings of the Brugada syndrome. These patients should be referred to an electrophysiologist for placement of an internal cardioverter-defibrillator, the only proven effective therapy. This patient, however, was not so fortunate. The ECG abnormality here was not recognized, and the patient was discharged after a brief laboratory workup for lightheadedness. One week later the patient had a cardiac arrest and died.

188. **SR, prolonged QT-interval suggestive of hypocalcemia.** The QT-interval is prolonged (QT = 468 msec, QTc = 550 msec). The differential diagnosis of QT-interval prolongation includes hypokalemia, hypomagnesemia, hypocalcemia, acute myocardial ischemia, elevated intracranial pressure, drugs with sodium channel blocking effects, hypothermia, and congenital prolonged QT syndrome. With the exceptions of only hypocalcemia and hypothermia, all of the listed conditions prolong the QT-interval by specifically prolonging the *T-wave*. Hypocalcemia and hypothermia prolong the QT-interval by specifically prolonging the *ST-segment*. In this case, the T-wave appears normal in size, whereas the ST-segment appears prolonged. Given the absence of bradycardia, Osborne waves, or tremor artifact, hypothermia is less likely and the diagnosis of hypocalcemia is

made. This patient had a recurrent seizure associated with torsade de pointes in the emergency department and was given intravenous calcium empirically based on the ECG findings, with excellent results. Afterwards, the initial serum calcium result was found to be 4.8 mg/dL (normal 8.8–10.2 mg/dL). See figure below.

This figure corresponds to case #188. QT-interval prolongation

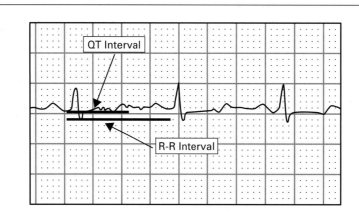

Comparison of QT-interval to the R-R interval. In this case, the QT-interval is greater than one-half the accompanying R-R interval. Thus, the QT interval is prolonged for this rate.

189. **SB, rate 46, BER, HLVV and Q-waves in lateral leads suggestive of hypertrophic cardiomyopathy.** Large amplitude QRS complexes are present in the precordial leads. In young patients, this is referred to as high left ventricular voltage (HLVV), as the diagnosis of LVH is usually reserved for patients >40 years of age. Mild STE is present in the mid precordial leads, a common finding in young men which may be diagnosed as BER when other findings suggestive of acute MI (evolving changes, reciprocal ST segment depression, convex-upwards STE, STE in other leads, etc.) are absent. A relatively tall R-wave is present in lead V1, defined when the R-wave approximates the size of or is larger than the S-wave. The differential diagnosis for this finding includes WPW, posterior MI, complete or incomplete RBBB, ventricular ectopy, RVH, acute right ventricular dilatation (right ventricular "strain," e.g. massive pulmonary embolism), hypertrophic cardiomyopathy, progressive muscular dystrophy, dextrocardia, and misplaced precordial leads. Amongst this list, hypertrophic cardiomyopathy (HCM) should be considered most strongly, especially in the presence of HLVV, a typical finding for patients with HCM. Further suggesting this diagnosis is the presence of deep narrow Q-waves in lateral leads V5–V6 and (especially) in leads I and aVL. These Q-waves are often misdiagnosed as evidence of an old lateral MI, but these are not infarction-related Q-waves because they are too narrow (<40 msec.). This combination of deep narrow Q-waves in the lateral leads plus HLVV, especially in a young patient with recent syncope, warrants immediate consideration of HCM. This patient had an urgent Doppler echocardiogram which confirmed the diagnosis, and he was treated with beta-blocker medications. See figure opposite.

190. **VT versus ST with aberrant conduction, rate 143.** This is a difficult rhythm in that it is uncertain whether the small upward deflections between the larger QRS complexes in lead V1 represent P-waves, retrograde atrial beats, or T-waves. T-waves of this size would be somewhat unusual. Even excluding T-waves, however, the diagnosis between VT (with retrograde atrial beats) versus ST with aberrant conduction remains uncertain. One clue, however, lies in the duration of the QRS complex. It is unusual for VT to cause such a wide (>200 msec. here) QRS complex. This magnitude of QRS widening is more likely to be caused by a metabolic abnormality associated with aberrant conduction, such as severe hyperkalemia. A trial of intravenous sodium bicarbonate boluses was given

This figure corresponds to case #189

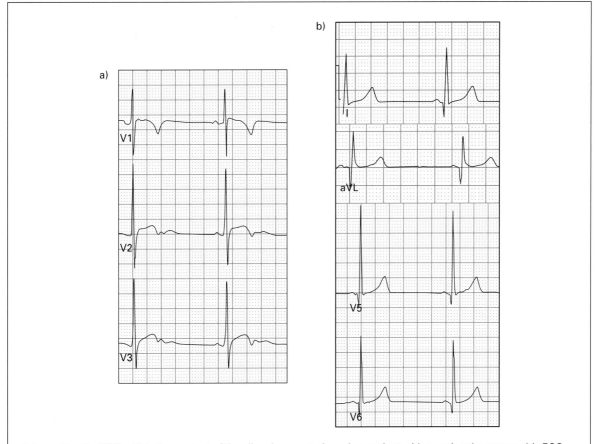

Interpreting the ECG within the context of the clincal presentation—in a patient with exertional syncope, this ECG should strongly suggest hypertrophic cardiomyopathy. a) Note the prominent R-waves in leads V1 to V3. b) The deep narrow Q-waves in the lateral leads are very suggestive of HCM.

and this resulted in a slight slowing of the rate and narrowing of the QRS complexes, confirming hyperkalemia. The serum potassium level was later found to be 9.1 mEq/L (normal 3.5–5.3 mEq/L). One other diagnosis deserves consideration here as well. ST with marked STE due to acute MI can also sometimes produce very wide, tall complexes in the anterior leads due to fusion of the elevated ST-segments with the QRS complex. However, the rightward axis and morphology of the QRS complexes in lead I rules this possibility out. In order for rightward axis to be attributed to MI, there must be large Q-waves in lead I. However, the QRS complexes in lead I are far too wide to be considered large Q-waves. Furthermore, there are no leads that demonstrate reciprocal ST-segment depression. Therefore, acute anterior MI is unlikely. See figure on p. 198.

191. **SR, rate 90, WPW, frequent PVCs in a pattern of ventricular bigeminy, anterior ischemia versus acute posterior MI.** The first QRS complex and every other complex following that is preceded by a P-wave with a short PR-interval, and delta-waves are present in these complexes (best seen in the lateral leads), consistent with underlying WPW. These intrinsic complexes alternate with PVCs, which occur in a pattern of bigeminy. Conduction through the accessory pathway of WPW commonly produces Q-waves in the inferior leads and a leftward axis.

Text continues on p. 199.

This figure corresponds to case #190

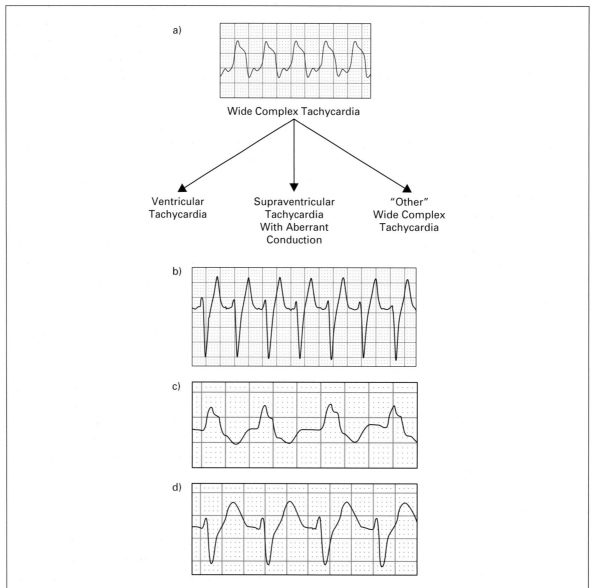

a) Wide Complex Tachycardia

Ventricular Tachycardia

Supraventricular Tachycardia With Aberrant Conduction

"Other" Wide Complex Tachycardia

b)

c)

d)

a) The traditional differential diagnosis of the wide complex tachycardia includes ventricular tachycardia and supraventricular tachycardia with aberrant ventricular conduction. Certainly, patient management is determined by the clinical presentation with unstable patients requiring more urgent, more aggressive therapies. Yet one particular consideration which must be made in this situation is the consideration of the "other" wide QRS complex tachycardias. These "other" entities include sinus tachycardia with either pre-existing or rate-related bundle branch block, metabolic events such as hyperkalemia, or poisonings such as excessive exposure to sodium-channel blocking agents. b) Sinus tachycardia with either pre-existing or rate-related bundle branch block. c) Metabolic events such as hyperkalemia. d) Poisonings such as excessive exposure to sodium channel blocking agents. P-waves are often absent in c) and d), making the distinction difficult without clinical information.

This should not be interpreted as evidence of a prior inferior MI; this is just a normal variant of WPW. Another pseudo-infarction pattern that is common with WPW is the presence of tall R-waves in the right precordial leads which mimic a prior posterior MI. Deep ST-segment depression in these leads, however, is *not* a normal variant and should be assumed to be an indication of acute anterior ischemia or acute posterior MI. Posterior leads were used in this case to exclude acute posterior MI. The ST-segment depression resolved after administration of nitroglycerin, and the patient then underwent unsuccessful PCI of a critical occlusion in the LAD artery. Cardiac bypass surgery was performed and he did well.

192. **Atrial fibrillation with third degree AV block and accelerated idioventricular rhythm, ventricular rate 64, rhythm suggestive of digoxin toxicity.** The underlying atrial activity appears to be fibrillation. Atrial fibrillation should be associated with an irregular ventricular response. In this case, however, the ventricular complexes are regular. This can only occur if all of the atrial impulses are blocked before reaching the ventricle, and an alternative focus in the AV junction or ventricle has assumed pacemaking activity. In other words, there is a third degree (complete) AV block and an escape rhythm is emanating from the AV junction or the ventricle. The morphology of the QRS complexes—wide, taller "left rabbit ear" in lead V1, rightward axis—is more consistent with a ventricular escape rhythm ("idioventricular" rhythm). Because the rate is faster than the normal ventricular escape rate (20–40 beats/minute), the designation *accelerated* idioventricular rhythm is used. Atrial fibrillation with complete heart block and slow escape rhythm is classic for digoxin toxicity. In this case, the patient did in fact have digoxin toxicity (serum level 4.8 ng/mL; normal 0.5–2.2 ng/mL).

193. **SR, rate 61, LAFB, T-wave abnormality suggestive of Wellens' syndrome.** Wellens' syndrome refers to an electrocardiographic T-wave abnormality in leads V2–V4 which has been described as highly specific for a critical occlusion in the proximal LAD artery.[6] The T-waves can demonstrate either deep inversions or a biphasic appearance. The T-wave abnormality persists even in the pain-free state. These patients are best managed with PCI, without which they are at high risk for extensive anterior wall MI or death within weeks. This patient's ECG demonstrates a subtle but definite biphasic appearance of the T-waves (terminal inversion of the T-waves) in leads V2–V4. This was interpreted as just a "non-specific T-wave abnormality," and the patient was discharged after an unremarkable laboratory workup. Two weeks later the patient had a massive MI. The infarct-related artery was, not surprisingly, the LAD.

194. **SR with first degree AV block, rate 60, LVH, short QT-interval, consider hypercalcemia.** The major diagnostic finding in this case is the short QT-interval (QT = 340 msec.; QTc = 330 msec.). A short QT-interval (QTc <400 msec) should prompt consideration of hypercalcemia and digoxin toxicity. More marked shortening of the QT-interval (QTc <300 msec) has recently been described in a genetic condition associated with sudden cardiac death.[11] The presentation and ECG in this case are strongly suggestive of hypercalcemia. Significant digoxin toxicity is unlikely given the absence of advanced AV blocks, bradycardias, or slurring of the downstroke of the QRS complexes ("digoxin effect"). The serum calcium level here was 16.0 mg/dL (normal 9.0–10.6 mg/dL).

195. **ST with second degree AV block and 2:1 AV conduction, rate 50, LBBB.** P-waves occur at a rate of 100 beats/minute, but many are hidden, or "buried," within T-waves. The hidden P-waves were missed by the treating physicians, and the ECG was misdiagnosed as sinus bradycardia. The patient was admitted for observation, but on the night of admission she progressed to third degree AV block and developed hemodynamic decompensation. The physicians involved then re-reviewed this original ECG and realized the mistake. A clue to the hidden P-waves lies in the morphology of the T-waves: the third T-wave has a "camel-hump" appearance, and the remainder have a slightly peaked apex. These two findings should always prompt consideration of buried P-waves. One then notices that these peaks map out with the other P-waves and therefore are actually buried atrial beats. Two P-waves are present for each QRS, and therefore the diagnosis of second degree AV block with 2:1 AV

conduction is made. When 2:1 AV conduction is present, more specific designation as Mobitz I or Mobitz II cannot be made.

196. **ST, rate 118, low voltage, consider pericardial effusion.** Low voltage is diagnosed when the QRS complex amplitudes in all of the limb leads are <5 mm in size *or* when the QRS complex amplitudes in all of the precordial leads are <10 mm in size. The differential diagnosis of low voltage includes myxedema, large pericardial effusion, large pleural effusion, end-stage cardiomyopathy, severe chronic obstructive pulmonary disease, severe obesity, infiltrative myocardial diseases, constrictive pericarditis, and prior massive MI. When the low voltage is known to be new, and especially in the presence of tachycardia, pericardial effusion should strongly be considered. This patient was initially diagnosed as having an acute inferior and lateral MI, a mistake that easily occurs when the end of the PR-segment is used as the isoelectric portion of the ECG. This results in the incorrect impression that STE is present. In reality, when the T-P segment is correctly used as the isoelectric portion of the ECG, one realizes that there is no STE (see figure below). Rather, there is mild PR-segment depression in some leads. PR-segment depression may occur in the setting of atrial infarction, abnormal atrial repolarization, pericarditis (when STE is present), or it may simply be a normal variant. The key point here is that there is no STE. Because of the misdiagnosis, the patient received anticoagulant therapy and was taken for PCI where it was found that the patient had a large pericardial effusion. The effusion became hemorrhagic and pericardial tamponade developed. The patient was found to have no coronary occlusions, and the effusion was later attributed to pericardial metastases from his cancer.

This figure corresponds to case #196. A comparison of the PR-segment, ST-segment, and electrocardiographic baseline

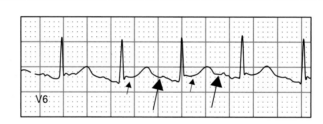

The small arrows point to the ST-segments and the large arrows at the T-P segments. Using the T-P segments, one notices that there is no ST segment elevation, only PR-segment depression.

197. **SR, rate 70, anterolateral MI of undetermined age with persistent STE suggesting acute MI versus ventricular aneurysm.** Large Q-waves are present in anterolateral leads V1–V5, I, and aVL indicative of MI. The additional presence of STE in leads V2–V5 are strongly suggestive that the MI is acute. However, given the large size of this apparent acute MI, the absence of *any* reciprocal ST-segment changes in the limb leads is unusual. Although reciprocal changes are not always present in the setting of an acute MI, their absence in the setting of a large anterior MI should at least call the diagnosis into some question. The additional history that the patient has had a prior MI should prompt consideration of the possibility of a ventricular aneurysm. Ventricular aneurysms are associated with persistent and long-standing STE with Q-waves after MI, but unlike the acute MI they generally are not associated with any reciprocal ST-segment changes. Because of the uncertainty in the diagnosis for this patient, fibrinolytics were withheld pending serial ECGs (which showed no evolving ST-segment or T-wave changes) and emergent echocardiography. This patient did, in fact, prove to have an anterior wall ventricular aneurysm and ruled out for acute cardiac ischemia.

198. **Accelerated idioventricular rhythm, rate 114.** This is a regular, wide QRS complex tachydysrhythmia without apparent P-waves. Although the first assumption might be VT, the rate is too slow: the diagnosis of VT should be reserved for ventricular rhythms >120 beats/minute. The rhythm is therefore referred to as AIVR. Slower rhythms that appear regular with wide QRS complexes and without P-waves are most commonly caused by reperfusion dysrhythmias (AIVR), severe hyperkalemia, and toxicities from sodium-channel blocking medications (including cyclic antidepressants, cocaine, etc.). If the diagnosis of VT is inappropriately made in any of these circumstances and the patient is treated with typical ventricular antidysrhythmics, the consequences can be fatal because many of these medications (e.g. lidocaine, procainamide, amiodarone) also have sodium-channel blocking effects. This patient, unfortunately, was misdiagnosed as having VT and treated with a bolus of intravenous lidocaine. Immediately after the bolus, the patient developed asystole and died. It was later discovered that the patient had a markedly elevated serum potassium level (he had developed renal failure and hyperkalemia because of systemic illness). Hyperkalemia is known to produce sodium channel dysfunction, a condition which can be exacerbated to deadly proportions when ventricular antidysrhythmics are added.[12]

199. **SB with isorhythmic AV dissociation and third degree AV block, AV junctional escape rhythm, rate 38, PRWP.** The QRS complexes occur at a rate of 38 beats/minute. P-waves are present as well at approximately the same rate and are best found in the latter half of the rhythm strip. However, tracing the P-waves backwards to the beginning of the ECG, it appears that some of the P-waves are hidden within the QRS complexes, and additionally the PR-interval in the 4th complex is too short for the P-wave to have been conducted. This implies that the atria and ventricles are operating independently—AV dissociation. When the atria and ventricles are dissociated but beating at nearly the same rate, the term "isorhythmic AV dissociation" is often used. Because the QRS complexes are perfectly regular, it is presumed that none of the P-waves are being conducted—third degree (complete) AV heart block. The escape rhythm is narrow and therefore the result of an AV junctional escape.

200. **Atrial rhythm with AV dissociation and third degree AV block, ventricular escape rhythm, rate 35, prominent T-waves suggestive of hyperkalemia.** Subtle atrial activity can be found in the rhythm strip at a rate of 80 beats/minute. SR produces upright P-waves in leads I, II, III, and aVF; and inverted P-waves in lead aVR. It is difficult to accurately assess the P-wave morphology in the majority of the limb leads therefore a simple diagnosis of atrial rhythm is made. The atrial beats are dissociated from the ventricular beats and the ventricular complexes occur regularly, implying AV dissociation with complete heart block. The QRS complexes are wide and occur at a typical ventricular escape rate (20–40 beats/minute). Prominent T-waves with mild peaking, especially in the precordial leads, suggests hyperkalemia. The patient's serum potassium level was 8.5 mEq/L (normal 3.5–5.3 mEq/L). Hyperkalemia produces all of the abnormalities noted in this ECG: prominent T-waves, flattening of the P-waves, AV blocks, and ventricular rhythms. This patient was originally treated with atropine and transcutaneous pacing but neither were effective. When the hyperkalemia was discovered, intravenous calcium, sodium bicarbonate, and insulin were administered with complete resolution of *all* abnormalities.

References

1. Sgarbossa EB, Pinski SL, Barbagelata A, *et al.* Electrocardiographic diagnosis of evolving acute myocardial infarction in the presence of left bundle-branch block, GUSTO-1 (Global Utilization of Streptokinase and Tissue Plasminogen Activator for Occluded Coronary Arteries) Investigators. *N Engl J Med* 1996;**334**:481–7.
2. Marriott HJL. *Marriott's Manual of Electrocardiography*. Orlando, FL: Trinity Press, 1995; p. 141.
3. Kosuge M, Kimura K, Ishikawa T, *et al.* Electrocardiographic differentiation between acute pulmonary embolism and acute coronary syndromes on the basis of negative T waves. *Am J Cardiol* 2007;**99**:817–21.
4. Brugada P, Brugada J. Right bundle branch block, persistent ST-segment elevation and sudden cardiac death: A distinct clinical and electrocardiograhic syndrome. *J Am Coll Cardiol* 1992;**20**:1391–6.
5. Marriott HJL. *Pearls and Pitfalls in Electrocardiography*, 2nd edn. Baltimore, MD: Williams & Wilkins, 1998.
6. De Zwann C, Bar FW, Wellens HJJ. Characteristic electrocardiographic pattern indicating a critical stenosis high in left anterior descending coronary artery in patients admitted because of impending myocardial infarction. *Am Heart J* 1982;**103**:730–6.

7. Antzelevitch C, Brugada P, Bordrefe M, *et al.* Brugada syndrome—report of the Second Consensus Conference. *Circulation* 2005;**111**:659–70.

8. Marriott HJL. *Emergency Electrocardiography*. Naples, FL: Trinity Press, 1997.

9. Sovari AA, Farokhi F, Kocheril AG. Inverted U wave, a specific electrocardiographic sign of cardiac ischemia. *Am J Emerg Med* 2007;**25**:235–7.

10. Gerson MC, McHenry PL. Resting U wave inversion as a marker of stenosis of the left anterior descending coronary artery. *Am J Med* 1980;**69**:545–50.

11. Gaita F, Giustetto C, Bianchi F, *et al.* Short QT syndrome. A familial cause of sudden death. *Circulation* 2003;**108**:965–70.

12. McLean SA, Paul ID, Spector PS. Lidocaine-induced conduction disturbance in patients with systemic hyperkalemia. *Ann Emerg Med* 2000;**36**:615–27.

Appendix A

Differential diagnoses

Diffuse ST-segment elevation
Large AMI, acute pericarditis, benign early repolarization, left ventricular hypertrophy, coronary vasospasm

Increased QRS-interval
Hypothermia, hyperkalemia, WPW, aberrant intraventricular conduction (e.g. bundle branch block), ventricular ectopy, electronic pacemakers, medications (extensive list), left ventricular hypertrophy, non-specific intraventricular delay (if none of the above are diagnosed)

Increased QT-interval (and QTc-interval)
Hypokalemia,* hypomagnesemia, hypocalcemia, acute myocardial ischemia, elevated intracranial pressure, drugs with sodium channel blocking effects (e.g. cyclic antidepressants, quinidine, etc.), hypothermia, and congenital prolonged QT syndrome

*Hypokalemia is included in this differential diagnosis for consideration; however, the actual QT-interval is normal; the QT-interval *appears* prolonged because of the presence of fusion of the T-wave with a U-wave (a "T-U fusion complex")

Leftward axis
LAFB, LBBB, inferior myocardial infarction (if Q-waves are present), left ventricular hypertrophy, ventricular ectopy, electronic pacemakers, and Wolff-Parkinson-White syndrome

Low voltage
Myxedema, large pericardial effusion, large pleural effusion, end-stage cardiomyopathy, severe chronic obstructive pulmonary disease, severe obesity, infiltrative myocardial diseases, constrictive pericarditis, and prior massive MI

Poor R-wave progression (PRWP)
Prior anteroseptal MI, LVH, abnormally high placement of the mid-precordial electrodes, or may simply be a normal variant

Prominent R-wave in lead V1
WPW, posterior MI, RBBB (or incomplete RBBB), ventricular ectopy, RVH, acute right ventricular dilatation (right ventricular "strain," e.g. massive pulmonary embolism), hypertrophic cardiomyopathy, progressive muscular dystrophy, dextrocardia, and misplaced precordial electrodes. The prominent R-wave in lead V1 (defined as an R:S ratio =1) exists as a normal variant in only rare instances.

Prominent T-wave
Acute myocardial ischemia, hyperkalemia, acute pericarditis, LVH, BER, bundle branch block, and pre-excitation syndromes

Rightward axis
LPFB, lateral myocardial infarction (if Q-waves are present), right ventricular hypertrophy, acute (e.g. pulmonary embolism) and chronic (e.g. emphysema) lung disease, ventricular ectopy, hyperkalemia, overdoses of sodium channel

blocking drugs (e.g. cyclic antidepressants), and misplaced leads. Normal young or slender adults with a horizontally positioned heart can also demonstrate a rightward QRS axis on the ECG.

ST-segment elevation in lead V1

LVH, LBBB, acute anteroseptal MI, acute right ventricular MI, Brugada syndrome, pulmonary embolism

Tachydysrhythmias

Narrow-complex regular rhythm: ST, SVT, atrial flutter

Narrow-complex irregular rhythm: atrial fibrillation, atrial flutter with variable block, MAT

Wide-complex regular rhythm: VT, ST with aberrant conduction, SVT with aberrant conduction, atrial flutter with aberrant conduction

Wide-complex irregular rhythm: atrial fibrillation with aberrant conduction (e.g. bundle branch block), atrial flutter with variable block and aberrant conduction, MAT with aberrant conduction, atrial fibrillation with WPW, polymorphic ventricular tachycardia

Appendix B

Commonly used abbreviations

AIVR	accelerated idioventricular rhythm
AMI	acute myocardial infarction
AV	atrioventricular
BER	benign early repolarization
HCM	hypertrophic cardiomyopathy
HLVV	high left ventricular voltage
IVCD	intraventricular conduction delay
LAD	left anterior descending (artery)
LAE	left atrial enlargement
LAFB	left anterior fascicular block
LBBB	left bundle branch block
LMCA	left main coronary artery
LPFB	left posterior fascicular block
LVH	left ventricular hypertrophy
MAT	multifocal atrial activity
MI	myocardial infarction
PAC	premature atrial contraction
PAT	paroxysmal atrial tachycardia
PCI	percutaneous intervention (refers to balloon angioplasty or stent placement)
PJC	premature junctional complex
PMI	posterior myocardial infarction
PVC	premature ventricular contraction
PRWP	poor R-wave progression
PS	pacemaker "spike"
QTc	corrected QT-interval
RBBB	right bundle branch block
RCA	right coronary artery
RV	right ventricle/right ventricular
RVH	right ventricular hypertrophy
SB	sinus bradycardia
SR	sinus rhythm
ST	sinus tachycardia
STE	ST-segment elevation
SVT	supraventricular tachycardia
TDP	torsade de pointes
VT	ventricular tachycardia
WCT	wide QRS complex tachycardia
WPW	Wolff-Parkinson-White syndrome

Index

Page numbers in **bold** refer to those pages on which electrocardiographs appear

aberrant conduction
  atrial fibrillation **127**, 172
  multifocal atrial tachycardia **122**, 168
  occasional **66**, 107, **108**
  see also ventricular conduction, aberrant
accelerated atrioventricular junctional rhythm **8**, **15**, 20, 24, **25**
  sinus rhythm with AV dissociation and third degree AV block **9**, 20, **22**
  SR with AV dissociation and third degree AV block **153**, 191
accelerated atrioventricular junctional tachycardia **51**, 95, **152**, 191
accelerated idioventricular rhythm **7**, **14**, 20, 23–4, **128**, **133**, 173, 177
  atrial fibrillation with third degree AV block **159**, 199
  versus sinoventricular rhythm **61**, 104
  wide QRS complex tachycardia **144**, 185
  wide QRS complex tachydysrhythmia **162**, 201
accelerated sinoventricular rhythm **61**, 104
anteroseptal ischemia **4**, 18
artifact, atrial fibrillation **3**, 17
atrial fibrillation **3**, 17
  aberrant ventricular conduction **15**, 24, **57**, 100, **101**
  acute anterior-lateral MI **53**, 97
  bifascicular block **139**, 181
  diffuse ischemia **54**, 97
  intraventricular conduction delay **133**, 177
  LBBB **145**, 185
  LVH **134**, 178
  occasional aberrant conduction **66**, 107, **108**
  with PVCs **141**, 183
  with rapid ventricular response **44**, 89, **90**
  with third degree AV block **159**, 199
  ventricular rate increase **127**, **128**, 172, 173
  WPW syndrome **59–60**, 102–3, **123**, 168–9
    ventricular rate increase **136**, 178–9
atrial flutter
  with 2:1 AV conduction **129**, **145**, **150**, 174–5, 185, 189–90
  with 4:1 atrioventricular conduction **6**, 19
  with variable AV conduction **121**, 166–7
atrial tachycardia
  AV conduction 2:1 **135**, 178
  ectopic **149**, 189
  with second degree AV block **123**, **151**, 168, 190–1
  see also multifocal atrial tachycardia (MAT)
atrioventricular (AV) block
  first degree with SB **154**, 193
  first degree with SR **8**, 20
    acute anterior-lateral MI **57**, 100
    acute inferior MI **146**, 185–6
    acute inferior-lateral MI **68**, 108, **110**
    bifascicular block **67**, 108, **109**, **126**, 170–1
    IVCD **124**, 169, **170**
    LBBB **119**, 164, 165
    LVH **160**, 199
    premature AV junctional complexes **67**, 107–8, **109**
  first degree with ST **36**, **42**, 83, 88

high-grade **11**, 23
  with SR **39**, 86
second degree with SR **10**, **11**, 20, **21**, 23, **41**, 88
  benign early repolarization **45**, 90
  LRRR **48**, 93, **94**
  LVH with repolarization abnormality **31**, 79
  non-specific IVCD **39**, 86
  persistent juvenile T-wave **124**, 169
second degree with ST **37**, 83–4, **142**, 183–4
  AV conduction 2:1 **161**, 199–200
  lateral ischemia **149**, 189
  PJCs and PVCs **151**, 190
third degree
  with atrial fibrillation **159**, 199
  AV dissociation with ST **16**, 24, **136**, 179
  with ectopic atrial rhythm **163**, 201
  variable with ectopic atrial tachycardia **149**, 189
  see also atrioventricular (AV) dissociation, with SR and third degree AV block; Mobitz atrioventricular blocks
atrioventricular (AV) conduction
  2:1 with atrial flutter **129**, **145**, **150**, 174–5, 185, 189–90
  2:1 with atrial tachycardia **135**, 178
  2:1 with ST and second degree AV block **161**, 199–200
  variable **121**, 166–7
atrioventricular (AV) dissociation
  with ectopic atrial rhythm **163**, 201
  isorhythmic with SB **163**, 201
  with SR **153**, 192
    ventricular escape rhythm **154**, 192
  with SR and third degree AV block **9**, 20, **22**
    AV junctional escape rhythm **130**, **148**, **153**, 175, 187–8, 191
  with ST and third degree AV block **16**, 24
    junctional escape rhythm **136**, 179
atrioventricular (AV) junctional escape rhythm **16**, 24
  RBBB **32**, 80, **81**, **153**, 192
  with SB **34**, 82
  SR with AV dissociation and third degree AV block **148**, 187–8
atrioventricular (AV) junctional rhythm **65**, 105
  accelerated **130**, 175
  anteroseptal MI **56**, 99, **100**

benign early repolarization (BER) **45**, 90
  with SB **158**, 196, **197**
  with SR **69**, **73**, 110, **111**, 113
bifascicular block
  accelerated junctional tachycardia **51**, 95
  atrial fibrillation **127**, **139**, 172, 181
  SR
    first degree AV block **67**, 107–8, **109**, **126**, 170–1
    third degree AV block **130**, 175
Brugada syndrome **126**, 171, **172**
  STE **140**, 181–2
    with SR and incomplete RBBB **157**, 195
    with ST and incomplete RBBB **150**, 189

cardiac ischemia, abnormal T waves **33**, 80, 82
case histories **3–16**
coronary artery *see* left main coronary artery (LMCA) occlusion

digitalis effect, SR with first degree AV block **38**, 85
digoxin toxicity
    atrial fibrillation with third degree AV block **159**, 199
    variable AV block with ectopic atrial tachycardia **149**, 189

ectopic atrial rhythm **33**, 82
    with AV dissociation **163**, 201

high left ventricular voltage (HLVV)
    SB **127**, 172–3
        benign early repolarization **158**, 196, **197**
    SR **43**, 88, **89**
        acute septal MI **43**, 88–9
hypercalcemia, short QT-interval **160**, 199
hyperkalemia
    accelerated idioventricular rhythm **61**, 104
    atrial fibrillation **57**, 100, **101**
    intraventricular conduction delay **124**, 169, **170**
    ST **147**, 187
    T-wave abnormality **30**, **45**, **49**, 78, 90, **91**, 95
        atrial fibrillation **134**, 178
        peaked **61**, 104
        prominent **153**, **163**, 191, 201
    versus VT **75**, 114
hypertrophic cardiomyopathy, Q-wave abnormalities **127**, **158**,
        172–3, 196, **197**
hypocalcemia, prolonged QT-interval **148**, 188–9
    with SR **157**, 195–6
hypokalemia
    with SR and prolonged QT-interval **135**, 178
    T-wave abnormality **41**, **52**, 88, 96–7
    U-wave abnormality **30**, 78, **125**, **132**, 170, **171**, 176
        with SR **135**, 178
hypothermia, Osborne waves **40**, **50**, 87, 95, **96**

intracranial hemorrhage, T-wave abnormality **33**, **48**, 80, 82, 92,
        93
intraventricular conduction delay (IVCD)
    atrial fibrillation **133**, 177
        with PVCs **141**, 183
    hyperkalemia **124**, 169, **170**
    multifocal atrial tachycardia **122**, 168
    non-specific **47**, 92
        with ST **65**, 105–6, **107**, **156**, 194
    SB with first degree AV block **154**, 193
    SR
        first degree AV block **38**, **49**, 85, 95
        second degree AV block **39**, 86
    ST with first degree AV block **45**, 90, **91**

junctional complex
    premature with aberrant conduction **8**, 20
    trigeminy **146**, **152**, 186–7, 191
junctional escape rhythm **130**, 175
J-waves *see* Osborne waves

left anterior fascicular block (LAFB) **67**, 108, **109**
    accelerated junctional tachycardia **51**, 95
    atrial fibrillation **44**, 89, **90**, **127**, **139**, 172, 181
    incomplete and accelerated AV junctional rhythm **130**,
        175
    SB **141**, 183
    SR **48**, 92, **93**, **122**, 168
        first degree AV block **67**, 107–8, **109**
        third degree AV block **130**, 175
        and T-wave abnormality **160**, 199
    ST **29**, 78, **150**, 189
        first degree AV block **42**, **45**, 88, 90, **91**

left atrial enlargement
    Brugada syndrome **140**, 181–2
    with SR **148**, 188–9
left bundle branch block (LBBB)
    atrial fibrillation **145**, 185
    SR **72**, 112, **122**, 168
        first degree AV block **119**, 164, 165
        ST-segment abnormality **139**, 181, **182**
    ST **58**, 100, **102**, **143**, 184–5
        second degree AV block **161**, 199–200
left main coronary artery (LMCA) occlusion
    AV junctional rhythm **56**, 99, **100**
    SR with HLVV **43**, 88–9
    ST
        first degree AV block **42**, 88
        infero-antero-lateral ischemia **36**, 83
left posterior fascicular block (LPFB)
    atrial flutter **121**, 166–7
    first degree AV block with SR **126**, 170–1
    incomplete with SVT **131**, 176
    with ST **63**, 105
left ventricular hypertrophy (LVH)
    atrial fibrillation **44**, 89, **90**, **134**, 178
    repolarization abnormality **31**, **59**, **75**, 79, 102, 114
    SB **152**, 191, **192**
        first degree AV block **147**, 187
    SR **37**, **48**, 84, 92, **93**
        first degree AV block **49**, 95, **146**, **160**, 185–6, 199
        high-grade AV block **39**, 86
    ST **37**, 83–4
leftward axis 203
low voltage 203
    electrical alternans **129**, 174
        pericardial effusion **129**, **138**, 174, 180
    pericardial effusion **161**, 200
        electrical alternans **129**, **138**, 174, 180
Lyme carditis **39**, 86

Mobitz I (Wenckebach) atrioventricular block **9**, 20, **21**, **39**,
        86
    with atrial tachycardia **151**, 190–1
    benign early repolarization **45**, 90
    incomplete RBBB **123**, 168
    lateral ischemia **149**, 189
    poor R-wave progression **132**, 177
    with SR **48**, **52**, 93, **94**, 97
Mobitz II atrioventricular block **11**, 23, **31**, 79
    with SR **41**, 88, **142**, 183
    with ST **37**, 83–4
    PJCs and PVCs **151**, 190
multifocal atrial tachycardia (MAT) **15**, 24, **25**, **47**, 92
    aberrantly conducted complexes **122**, 168
    wandering atrial pacemaker **32**, 80, **81**
myocardial infarction (MI)
    acute
        atrial fibrillation **145**, 185
        versus ventricular aneurysm **162**, 200
    acute anterior **36**, 83
        with SR **55**, 98
    acute anterior-lateral **53**, **56**, 97, 99
        SR with first degree AV block **57**, 100
        ST **121**, 166, **167**
    acute anterior-septal **128**, 173
    acute inferior **70–1**, 112
        SB with frequent PVCs **143**, 184
        SR **77**, 115
            first degree AV block **146**, 185–6
    acute inferior-anterior-lateral **122**, 168

acute inferior-anterior-septal **130**, 175
acute inferior-lateral **51**, 95–6
    atrial fibrillation **66**, 107, **108**
    SR with first degree AV block **68**, 108, **110**
acute inferior-posterior
    SB with frequent PVCs **144**, 185
    SR with AV dissociation and third degree AV block **148**, 187–8
acute inferior-posterior-lateral **38**, 85, **86**
    with ST **55**, 98, **99**
acute lateral **46**, 91
acute posterior **54**, 97
    atrial fibrillation **66**, 107, **108**
    SR **138**, 180
    SR with WPW syndrome **159**, 197, 199
    STE **76**, 115
acute right ventricular **146**, 185–6
    SR with AV dissociation and third degree AV block **148**, 187–8
acute septal **43**, 88–9
anterolateral with persistent STE **162**, 200
anteroseptal **51**, 95–6
    atrial tachycardia with Mobitz type I **151**, 190–1
    AV junctional rhythm **56**, 99, **100**
    SB with first degree AV block **154**, 193
    SR **120**, 165
    variable AV block with ectopic atrial tachycardia **149**, 189
inferior **36**, **53**, 83, 97
    atrial flutter with 2:1 AV conduction **145**, 185
    SB with first degree AV block **154**, 193
    with ST **137**, 179
    variable AV block with ectopic atrial tachycardia **149**, 189
inferior-anteroseptal **147**, 187
inferior-lateral **135**, 178
inferior-posterior-anterior **73**, 112–13
inferior-posterior-lateral **37**, **49**, 84, 95
lateral **44**, 89, **90**
right ventricular **37**, 84
septal **42**, 88
SR with first degree AV block **119**, 165
ST with STE **14**, 24
ST-segment abnormality **119**, **122**, 164, 168
    elevation **14**, **15**, 24, **25**
    with SR **139**, 181, **182**
myocardial ischemia
  anterior **42**, 88
    Mobitz type II **151**, 190
    SR with WPW syndrome **159**, 197, 199
    with ST **155**, 193
  anterolateral **35**, 82–3
    atrial fibrillation **127**, **139**, 172, 181
    with SR **64**, 105, **106**
  anteroseptal **35**, **40**, 82, 87
    with SB **76**, 115
  atrial fibrillation **54**, 97, **145**, 185
  diffuse with ST **155**, **156**, 193–4, 194–5
  inferior **40**, **42**, 87, 88
    with SR **64**, 105, **106**
    with ST **155**, 193
  infero-anterolateral **36**, 83, **126**, 170–1
  infero-anteroseptal **125**, 170
  inferolateral **56**, 99, **100**
    SR with AV dissociation **153**, 192
    SR with premature AV junctional complexes **146**, 186–7
  inverted U-waves **152**, 191, **192**
  lateral **70–1**, 112

Mobitz type I **149**, 189
  pericardial effusion **138**, 180
  variable AV block with ectopic atrial tachycardia **149**, 189
Mobitz I block **132**, **149**, 177, 189
multifocal atrial tachycardia **47**, 92
SR with first degree AV block **119**, 165
ST **37**, **63**, 83–4, 105
  incomplete RBBB **150**, 189
ST-segment abnormality **119**, **122**, 164, 168
  with SR **139**, 181, **182**
T-wave abnormality **40**, **48**, **52**, 87, 92, **93**, 96–7
  pulmonary embolism **137**, 179

Osborne waves
  hypothermia **40**, **50**, 87, 95, **96**
  sinus bradycardia **50**, 95, **96**

pacemaker
  paced rhythm (100%) **58**, 100, **101**
  ventricular paced rhythm **10**, 20, **22**
  wandering **53**, 97
    atrial **32**, 80, **81**
paroxysmal supraventricular tachycardia **5**, **13**, 19, 23
pericardial effusion, electrical alternans **140**, 182
pericarditis, acute
  ectopic atrial rhythm **33**, 82
  SR **50**, **68**, **74**, 95, 110, **111**, 113
    high left ventricular voltage **43**, 88, **89**
  ST **137**, 180
premature atrial contraction (PAC) **4**, 18
  atrial bigeminy pattern **47**, 92
  blocked **147**, 187
    SR with first degree AV block **154**, 193
  with SB **30**, 78
  with SR **4**, 18, **52**, 96–7, **131**, **134**, 175, 178
premature atrioventricular junctional complexes **67**, 107–8, **109**
  with SR **146**, 186–7
premature junctional complex (PJC)
  with aberrant conduction **8**, 20
  accelerated AV junctional tachycardia **152**, 191
  Mobitz type II **151**, 190
premature ventricular contraction (PVC) **4**, 18
  atrial fibrillation **128**, **141**, 173, 183
  Mobitz type II **151**, 190
  with R-on-T phenomenon **15**, 24, **25**
  with SB **10**, 23
    acute inferior-posterior MI **144**, 185
    ventricular bigeminy **143**, 184
  with SR **4**, 18, **122**, 168
    first degree AV block **38**, 85
  with ST **36**, **37**, 83–4
    diffuse ischemia **155**, 193–4
  variable AV block with ectopic atrial tachycardia **149**, 189
  wandering atrial pacemaker **32**, 80, **81**
pulmonary embolism
  inferior/anteroseptal myocardial ischemia **137**, 179
  SR with non-sustained VT **125**, 170
  ST
    incomplete RBBB **35**, 82
    inferior/anterior ischemia **155**, 193
    RVH **40**, 87

QRS complex
  narrow **3**, **6**, 17, 19
    accelerated atrioventricular junctional rhythm **8**, 20
    rhythm strip **12**, 23
  rapid **3**, 17
  varying **4**, 18

QRS complex (*cont'd*)
  wide **3**, **17**
    accelerated idioventricular rhythm **7**, 20
    with LVH **31**, 79
    VT **31**, 79, **80**
QRS-interval, increased 203
QT-interval
  increased 203
  prolonged **4**, 18
    accelerated junctional tachycardia **51**, 95
    hypocalcemia **148**, **157**, 188–9, 195–6
    hypokalemia **125**, **132**, **135**, 170, **171**, 176, 178
    SR **30**, **48**, 78, 92, **93**, **132**, 176
    ST **65**, 105–6, **107**, **155**, 193–4
    ST with biatrial enlargement **33**, 80, 82
    ST with first degree AV block **51**, 95–6
  short and hypercalcemia **160**, 199
quadrigeminy, PACs **30**, 78
Q-waves, hypertrophic cardiomyopathy **127**, **158**, 172–3, 196, **197**

repolarization, benign early **45**, 90
  with SB **158**, 196, **197**
  with SR **69**, **73**, 110, **111**, 113
right bundle branch block (RBBB)
  accelerated junctional tachycardia **51**, 95
  atrial fibrillation **44**, 89, **90**, **127**, **134**, **139**, 172, 178, 181
  atrial tachycardia **135**, 178
  AV junctional rhythm **32**, 80, **81**
    accelerated **130**, 175
    SR with AV dissociation **153**, 192
  incomplete **123**, 168
    accelerated AV junctional rhythm **130**, 175
    with SR **126**, 171, **172**
    with ST **150**, 189
    with STE **140**, **157**, 181–2, 195
    SVT **131**, 176
  intermittent **146**, 186–7
  Mobitz type II **142**, 183
  SB with first degree AV block **147**, 187
  SR
    first degree AV block **67**, 107–8, 108, **109**, **126**, 170–1
    third degree AV block **130**, 175
  ST **35**, **36**, 82, 83
    AV dissociation and third degree AV block **136**, 179
right ventricular hypertrophy (RVH), with ST **40**, 87
rightward axis 203–4
  ST **65**, 105–6, **107**
R-on-T phenomenon **15**, 24, **25**
R-wave, poor progression (PRWP) **64**, 105, **106**
  differential diagnosis 203
  Mobitz I block **132**, 177
  SB **141**, 183
    first degree AV block **154**, 193
  SR **74**, 114
  ST **137**, 179
R-wave, prominent 203

septal infarct **29**, 78
sinus bradycardia (SB) **6**, 19
  acute lateral MI **46**, 91
  anterolateral ischemia **35**, 82–3
  anteroseptal ischemia **76**, 115
  AV junctional escape beats **34**, 82
  benign early repolarization **158**, 196, **197**
  with first degree AV block **68**, 108, **110**
    blocked PACs **147**, **154**, 187, 193

frequent PACs **30**, 78
frequent PVCs **10**, 23, **143**, **144**, 184, 185
high left ventricular voltage **127**, 172–3
hypothermia **50**, 95, **96**
isorhythmic AV dissociation **163**, 201
LVH **152**, 191, **192**
poor R-wave progression **141**, 183
WPW syndrome **77**, 115
sinus rhythm (SR)
  aberrantly conducted complexes **73**, 112–13
  acute anterior MI **55**, 98
  acute inferior MI **70–1**, **77**, 112, 115
  acute inferior-posterior-lateral MI **38**, 85, **86**
  acute pericarditis **50**, **68**, **74**, 95, 110, **111**, 113
  acute posterior MI **138**, 180
  anterolateral MI **162**, 200
  anteroseptal MI **120**, 165
  artifact **72**, 112
  with AV dissociation **153**, 192
    ventricular escape rhythm **154**, 192
  with AV dissociation and third degree AV block **9**, 20, **22**
    accelerated AV junctional escape rhythm **153**, 191
    AV junctional escape rhythm **148**, 187–8
    junctional escape rhythm **130**, 175
  BER **69**, **73**, 110, **111**, 113
  with first degree AV block **8**, 20, **38**, **49**, **57**, 85, 95, 100
    acute anterior-lateral MI **57**, 100
    acute inferior MI **146**, 185–6
    bifascicular block **67**, 108, **109**, **126**, 170–1
    IVCD **124**, 169, **170**
    LBBB **119**, 164, 165
    LVH **160**, 199
    premature AV junctional complexes **67**, 107–8, **109**
  high left ventricular voltage **43**, 88, **89**
  with high-grade AV block **39**, 86
  hypokalemia **125**, **132**, 170, **171**, 176
    prolonged QT-interval **135**, 178
  incomplete RBBB **126**, 171, **172**
    with STE **140**, **157**, 181–2, 195
  J-wave abnormality **40**, 87
  LAFB
    and LVH **48**, 92, **93**
    T-wave abnormality **160**, 199
  LBBB **72**, 112
    ST-segment abnormality **139**, 181, **182**
  left atrial enlargement **148**, 188–9
  LVH **37**, 84
    repolarization changes **59**, **75**, 102, 114
  non-sustained VT **125**, 170
  with PAC
    atrial bigeminy pattern **47**, 92
    frequent **131**, 175
    occasional **134**, 178
    and PVC **4**, 18
  poor R-wave progression **64**, **74**, 105, **106**, 114
  premature atrial contractions **52**, 96–7
  premature AV junctional complexes **146**, 186–7
  premature ventricular contractions **122**, 168
  prolonged QT-interval **30**, 78
    hypocalcemia **157**, 195–6
  second degree AV block **9**, **11**, 20, **21**, 23, **31**, **41**, 79, 88
    HLVV **45**, 90
    LBBB **48**, 93, **94**
    LVH with repolarization abnormality **31**, 79
    non-specific IVCD **39**, 86
    persistent juvenile T-wave **124**, 169

poor R-wave progression **132**, 177
RBBB **52**, 97, **142**, 183
T-wave abnormality **41**, 88
peaked **61**, 104
persistent juvenile **34**, 82
wandering pacemaker **53**, 97
WPW syndrome **60**, 103, **159**, 197, 199
sinus tachycardia (ST) **5**, 19
acute anterior-lateral MI **56**, 99, **121**, 166, **167**
acute inferior-posterior-lateral MI **55**, 98, **99**
acute pericarditis **137**, 180
electrical alternans **140**, 182
with AV dissociation and third degree AV block **16**, 24
junctional escape rhythm **136**, 179
diffuse ischemia **156**, 194–5
with first degree AV block **36**, **42**, **51**, 83, 88, 95–6
LAFB **45**, 90, **91**
frequent PVCs **155**, 193–4
hyperkalemia **14**, 187
incomplete RBBB **35**, 82
with STE **150**, 189
inferior and anterior ischemia **155**, 193
inferior anterolateral ischemia **36**, 83
inferior MI **137**, 179
LBBB **58**, 100, **102**, **143**, 184–5
left anterior fascicular block **29**, 78
low voltage
electrical alternans **129**, **138**, 174, 180
pericardial effusion **161**, 200
LPFB **63**, 105
non-specific IVCD **156**, 194
prolonged QT-interval and biatrial enlargement **33**, 80, 82
right ventricular hypertrophy **40**, 87
rightward axis **65**, 105–6, **107**
with second degree AV block **37**, 83–4
aberrant ventricular conduction **142**, 183–4
AV conduction 2:1 **161**, 199–200
lateral ischemia **149**, 189
PJCs and PVCs **151**, 190
ST-segment elevation **14**, 24
versus VT **158**, 196–7, **198**
sodium channel blocking drug toxicity/overdose **65**, 105–6, **107**
SR with first degree AV block **126**, 170–1
ST with non-specific IVCD **156**, 194
versus VT **120**, 165–6
ST-segment abnormality
acute ischemia/MI **122**, 168
atrial fibrillation **145**, 185
with SR **139**, 181, **182**
SR with first degree AV block **119**, 164, 165
ST-segment depression (STD) **11**, 23
ST-segment elevation (STE) **15**, 24, **25**
acute posterior MI **76**, 115
anterolateral MI **162**, 200
Brugada syndrome **140**, 181–2
differential diagnosis 204
diffuse 203
incomplete RBBB **126**, 171, **172**
with ST **150**, 189
with ST **14**, 24, **150**, 189
supraventricular tachycardia (SVT) **54**, **62**, 98, 105
incomplete RBBB and LPFB **131**, 176
paroxysmal **5**, **13**, 19, 23

tachycardia
irregular **3**, 17
wide complex **10**, 20, **21**

see also atrial tachycardia; multifocal atrial tachycardia (MAT)
tachydysrhythmias 204
torsade de pointes **3**, **4**, 17, 18
polymorphic LMCA occlusion **46**, 91
T-waves
anteroseptal ischemia **35**, 82
diffuse cardiac ischemia **52**, 96–7
intracranial hemorrhage **33**, **48**, 80, 82, 92, **93**
flattening **50**, **53**, 95, **96**, 97
non-specific diffuse **73**, 112–13
hyperkalemia **30**, **45**, **49**, 78, 90, **91**, 95
atrial fibrillation **134**, 178
hypokalemia **41**, **52**, 88, 96–7
inferior/anteroseptal ischemia **40**, 87, **125**, **137**, 170, 179
pulmonary embolism **155**, 193
non-specific abnormality **127**, 172–3
peaked **61**, 104
persistent juvenile pattern **34**, 82
SR with second degree AV block **124**, 169
prominent
differential diagnosis 203
hyperkalemia **153**, **163**, 191, 201
Wellen's syndrome **141**, **160**, 183, 199

U-waves
hypokalemia **30**, 78, **125**, **132**, 170, **171**, 176
with SR **135**, 178
inverted **152**, 191, **192**

ventricular aneurysm
versus acute MI **162**, 200
SR **120**, 165
ventricular bigeminy
SB with frequent PVCs **143**, 184
SR with WPW syndrome **159**, 197, 199
ventricular conduction, aberrant **57**, 100, **101**
atrial fibrillation **15**, 24
ST with second degree AV block **142**, 183–4
ventricular escape rhythm
with ectopic atrial rhythm **163**, 201
SR with AV dissociation **154**, 192
ventricular fibrillation **14**, 23
PVC with R-on-T phenomenon **15**, 24
ventricular paced rhythm **10**, 20, **22**
ventricular pause **61**, 104
ventricular rate, increase with atrial fibrillation **127**, 172
ventricular tachycardia (VT) **7**, **14**, 20, **21**, 24, **44**, 89
versus hyperkalemia **75**, 114
non-sustained **125**, 170
polymorphic **4**, **15**, **16**, 18, 24, 25, **46**, 91
SB with frequent PVCs **10**, 23
versus sodium channel blocker toxicity **120**, 165–6
versus ST with aberrant conduction **158**, 196–7, **198**
wide QRS complex **31**, **48**, 79, **80**, 93, **94**

Wellen's syndrome **35**, **64**, 82–3, 105, **106**
T-wave abnormalities **141**, **160**, 183, 199
Wenckebach block *see* Mobitz I (Wenckebach) atrioventricular block
Wolff–Parkinson–White (WPW) syndrome
atrial fibrillation **3**, 17, **59–60**, 102–3
ventricular rate increase **123**, 168–9
SB **77**, 115
SR **60**, 103
with frequent PVCs **159**, 197, 199
with premature AV junctional complexes **146**, 186–7

ECGs for the Emergency Physician

Amal Mattu, University of Maryland Medical Center, Maryland, USA
William Brady, University of Virginia Medical Center, Charlottesville, USA

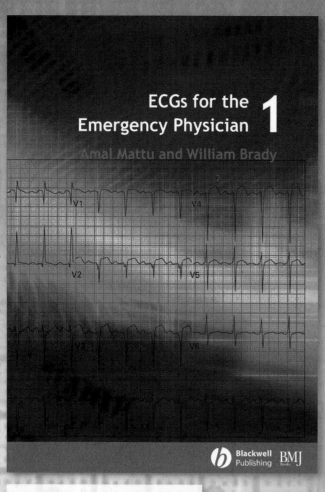

ECGs for the Emergency Physician **1**

Amal Mattu and William Brady

- Multiple examples of good quality ECGs for self education

- Designed especially for emergency medicine

- Categorised into level of difficulty

- Useful appendices to assist with diagnosis

ISBN 9780727916549 • Paperback
176 pages • September 2003

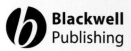

Blackwell
Publishing

To order or view a sample chapter visit
www.blackwellpublishing.com/9780727916549